Omega was founded in 1977 at a time when holistic health, psychological inquiry, world music and art, meditation, and new forms of spiritual practice were just budding in American culture. Omega was then just a small band of seekers searching for new answers to perennial questions about human health and happiness. The mission was as simple as it was large: to look everywhere for the most effective strategies and inspiring traditions that might help people bring more meaning and vitality into their lives.

Since then Omega has become the nation's largest holistic learning center. Every year more than 25,000 people attend workshops, retreats, and conferences in health, psychology, the arts, and spirituality on its eighty-acre campus in the countryside of Rhinebeck, New York, and at other sites around the country. While Omega has grown in size, its mission remains the same. Omega is not aligned with any particular healing method or spiritual tradition. Its programs feature all of the world's wisdom traditions and are committed to offering people an opportunity to explore their own path to better health, personal growth, and inner peace.

The name Omega was inspired by the writings of Pierre Teilhard de Chardin, a twentieth-century mystic and philosopher who used the word to describe the point within each one of us where our inner spiritual nature meets our outer worldly nature. Teilhard believed that the synthesis of these two domains presented the greatest challenge—and the greatest hope—for human evolution. Of his belief in the balance between world and spirit, Teilhard wrote, "I am going to broadcast the seed and let the wind carry it where it will."

Omega has taken on the task of helping spread that seed so that a better world for all of us can continue to take root and grow.

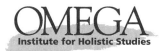

OMEGA
Institute for Holistic Studies

The Omega Institute
Mind, Body, Spirit Series

The Essentials of Yoga
Vitality and Wellness
Writing Your Authentic Self

AND COMING SOON . . .

Contemplative Living
The Power of Ritual
Bodywork Basics

An Omega Institute Mind, Body, Spirit Book

Writing Your Authentic Self

❖

Lois Guarino

A DELL TRADE PAPERBACK

A DELL TRADE PAPERBACK

Published by
Dell Publishing
a division of
Random House, Inc.
1540 Broadway
New York, New York 10036

Written by: Cheryl Jefferson
Series consulting editor: Robert Welsch
Series editor: Kathleen Jayes
Series manager: James Kullander
Literary representative: Ling Lucas, Nine Muses and Apollo Inc.

Dell books may be purchased for business or promotional use or for special sales.
For information please write to: Special Markets Department, Random House,
Inc., 1540 Broadway, New York, N.Y. 10036

DTP and the colophon are trademarks of Random House, Inc.

Library of Congress Cataloging in Publication Data
Guarino, Lois.
    Writing your authentic self / Lois Guarino
        p.   cm. — (The Omega Institute mind, body, spirit series)
    Includes index.
    ISBN 0-440-50871-1
    1. Self-actualization (Psychology)   2. Diaries—Authorship.
I. Sarley, Ila.   II. Title.   III. Series.
BF637.S4G83   1999
808'.06692—dc21   99-28318
                    CIP

Printed in the United States of America
Published simultaneously in Canada
September 1999

10 9 8 7 6 5 4 3 2 1

RRD

BOOK DESIGN BY JENNIFER ANN DADDIO

Omega Institute sends out heartfelt thanks and appreciation to staff members and teachers for their support and contribution in the preparation and publishing of this book.

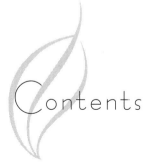Contents

Writing Your Authentic Self

Journal Writing— An Overview

A journal is a journey, your journey, and it can take you wherever you want to go. You don't have to be a writer. You don't have to fill your journal with literary efforts. You don't even have to write in complete sentences. All you have to do is be willing to start and see where it leads because a journal, like a journey, is about movement.

Just as a journey is about moving from one place to another, a journal is about interior movement on the path to finding your authentic self. The idea of an "authentic self" may seem foreign to you, but it's really quite simple. Your authentic self is the person composed of your most reliable instincts, truthful insights, trustworthy observations, and genuine feelings. It's also your talents and dreams, successes and failures. In short, your authentic self is everything you are and everything you have the potential to become. The purpose of a journal is to help you express this authenticity and to provide a deeply meaningful tool on your voyage of self-discovery. This book will show you the way.

In this chapter and the ones that follow, you will learn about a wide range of approaches, techniques, topics, and benefits associated with keeping a journal. You will be

"Learning is movement from moment to moment."
—J. KRISHNAMURTI, TEACHER AND PHILOSOPHER

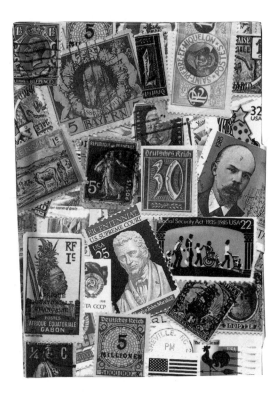

Cover of a travel journal
from the journal collection of the author

introduced to the work of teachers and the words of journal writers. You will discover that there is no right or wrong way to approach this subject and that there are as many varied, individual approaches to writing as there are people who write. This realization should liberate and reassure you, especially if you have never written before and worry that you must follow one particular style or format.

Whatever the case, use this book as a resource for finding your own voice and expressing it. The best way to begin is to explore the many options you'll find in these pages. Read them carefully and watch your reaction. Does one approach appeal to you more than another? Are there entries that move or inspire you? Do you feel motivated to pick up a pen and let your authentic self come through with some words of your own? If so, remember the following.

A Private Place

Your words belong to you. Unless you want to, you don't have to share them with anyone else. Your journal is a private place. It's a place to explore your creative and physical self and to examine feelings. Your environment, relationships, career, dreams, conversations, and community are also possible topics, as are the deeper issues like your place in life, your role in the universe, and your spirituality.

According to educator and well-known journal expert Christina Baldwin, these deeper issues are what distinguish a journal from a diary. Although the two words often are used interchangeably, there is a difference. A diary is a formal pattern of daily entries that catalog observations, activities, expenses, and the like. It is outwardly focused. By contrast, a journal is an inward journey, a record of internal life written consistently over a period of time but not necessarily day by day. It is a place where you can go one on one with your mind, where you can commune with rarely explored parts of yourself and where those parts can answer back. What are those other parts? Your intuition, your alter ego, your subconscious, and your spirit. We all have these answering voices, notes Baldwin, and through journal writing, we can access them.

But why should we? Paris-born Anaïs Nin, one of history's most famous journal writers, provided an answer in one of her entries.

"We write to heighten our . . . awareness of life . . . to taste life twice, in the moment and in retrospection . . . to transcend . . . life . . . to teach ourselves to speak with others, to record the journey into the labyrinth . . . expand our world, when we feel strangled, constricted, lonely . . . when I don't write I feel my world shrinking. I . . . lose my fire, my color."

Reasons for Keeping a Journal

Heightening your awareness is just one reason to keep a journal. There are many others. As you'll learn later in this book, you can use journals to study family history, as Alex Haley did in his research for the book *Roots*; to explain what it's like to live as an artist, as Andy Warhol did in *The Diaries of Andy Warhol*; or to understand why you're ill, like broadcaster Betty Rollins, who kept a journal on her fight against breast cancer. Whatever your reason for keeping a journal, you're in good company.

Ptolemy, Marco Polo, Samuel Pepys, Cleopatra, Abigail Adams, Anne Frank, and even fictional characters like Robinson Crusoe kept journals for the same reason you're thinking of doing it—to make sense of their lives. Along the way, each of these people discovered more about who they really were, even though at the time they may not have consciously known this is what they were doing.

Take Marco Polo. His intention was to chronicle his world travels, yet among the dates and descriptions are personal insights and observations of himself and others. As Marco Polo broadened his horizons, he also broadened his sense of self. Likewise, Cleopatra wrote of her great loves and passions, but she also used her journal to explore political strategies and assess the power of Rome. In her journal, Cleopatra's personal and professional politics cross-pollinated, defining her as a woman and a queen.

Obviously, journals work on many levels. You might think you're writing about your diet, but in among the notes on pounds you lost you might discover references to an old self-image you're ready to shed. Those entries on becoming a mother not only catalog the progress of your pregnancy, they may provide insights on the relationship between you and your parents, and so on.

The point is that a journal helps you communicate more clearly with yourself. As you will learn from the many journal writers and experts in this book, journal writing helps you achieve self-knowledge and self-healing. It guides you as you progress toward who you want to be. It's a way of making your dreams and goals more real. Ultimately, giving these elusive, intangible concepts a physical dimension is powerful medicine.

Powerful Medicine

Why medicine? Because writing a journal is healthy, says Sandra Thomas, Ph.D., R.N., a professor at the University of Tennessee College of Nursing and founder of the Women's Anger Study. Thomas notes that besides diffusing anger, a journal is a

"Develop the picture of your desire. Fill in as many details as you can without specifying how they shall come out."

—GEORGE WINSLOW PLUMMER, *CONSCIOUSLY CREATING CIRCUMSTANCES*

Susan Spritz Myers, founder and president of Living With
Your Heart, a life coaching service in Glencoe, Illinois,
has this to say about the power of the written word.

Q: Why do you ask your clients to write things down?

A: There are a couple of reasons. First, I find it helps people clear their minds of their daily schedule and the negative thoughts that swirl around in their heads. In coaching, we call those thoughts gremlins. Journaling is a wonderful outlet to release this stuff. Then people can begin to access the honesty within and get in touch with what is really important in their life. I believe in the power of the universe. If we can get completely clear and focused on our life goals, the universe will support us. I find writing is a wonderful vehicle to communicate directly with the universal power. I have seen amazing things happen when we hold the commitment of writing in a completely honest voice.

Q: Why continue once the vision is clear?

A: Because life happens and we get blocked or stopped on the journey. Writing gives you the opportunity to realize you are blocked, then you can look at the obstacles and think about how you want to progress. Introspective writing creates an awareness that is incredibly powerful and motivational.

Q: Can you give us an example?

A: I have one client, a forty-four-year-old woman, who wanted to save money, leave her corporate job, and sell a book. She'd had these same goals for years but never wrote them down. When we started working together, she began keeping a journal. Over a period of several months, she refined each of these goals in her journal entries. She identified a certain amount of money and how she might earn and save it, created a step-by-step plan for leaving her corporate job, and developed a specific idea for a book proposal as well as a time line for completing it. One year later, this client had eliminated her debt and built up her savings, negotiated a severance package with her employer, and completed a book proposal. The client is quite sure none of this would've happened without the power of the written word.

highly effective means of releasing stress and frustration. In addition, you can use your entries to respond to a health crisis, such as an illness, a physical challenge, or a body image problem. You also might want to change an old addictive habit, rebuild your self-esteem after a bad relationship, understand your father's death, or find out why, in any given situation, things turned out differently than you expected.

Whatever the case, journal writing helps you identify the issue and seek a solution. It does this by revealing recurrent patterns. A journal kept consistently over time can show you which situations regularly trigger certain emotions and behaviors. These can be behaviors you want to change or behaviors that are working just fine. If they're behaviors you want to change, your journal is the place where you can explore various options and evaluate potential outcomes. In other words, it is a safe place to try on the faces you're not quite ready to show to the world.

No matter what the world says, remember that your journal is not public

Protecting Your Privacy and Helping Others Cope with Fears About Your Journal

A journal is a powerful entity, writes Christina Baldwin, so powerful that it might frighten the people in your life. To help them cope with their fears about your entries and to maintain your privacy, Baldwin and other experts recommend the following:

+ Explain that everyone owns his or her own life story.

+ Remind others that your journal is about you, not them.

+ Assure them that your journal is private, that it will not be used for any questionable purpose.

+ If appropriate, describe the security measures you've taken and the code of honor you expect others to follow.

+ If you want to, share your journal with family members or friends.

+ Encourage the people you love to keep their own journals and assure them that you will respect their privacy.

property unless you choose to make it so. Therefore, in the interest of privacy, think about where you should keep it stored. Anaïs Nin kept her completed journals locked in a safety deposit box. You might use a locked drawer, briefcase, or fireproof metal box.

Any of these precautions might be appropriate depending on the circumstances. If you're leaving your employer or your spouse, working to get out of an abusive situation, have a brilliant scientific formula, or simply want to avoid prying eyes, plan security accordingly. Also, if you carry your journal out and about, you should insert a card inside with instructions on how it can be returned to you if it becomes lost. Include your name, address, phone number, and, if appropriate, offer a reward. If your journal is especially sensitive, you may want to substitute a post office box number for your name and address.

There's another issue to consider too. How accessible is your journal when you're not around? Have you told your housemates and family members how you feel about privacy? Will they respect your wishes? Are there other journal keepers in your home and is a code of honor strictly enforced?

And what happens to your journal when you die? Is there someone you can trust with it? Do you need to put written instructions about what's to be done and a key in your will? Do you want your journals assembled into a book, as novelist Virginia Woolf considered doing in this entry:

". . . what is to become of all these diaries . . . if I died, what would Leo make of them? He would be disinclined to burn them; he could not publish them. Well, he should make up a book from them, . . . I daresay there is a little book in them; if the scraps and scratchings were straightened out a little."

Or destroyed, like Mary Chestnut's mid-19th-century diaries that were immortalized in Ken Burns's *The Civil War*, an Emmy Award–winning documentary?

"Isabella has been reading my diaries. How we laugh at my sage ratiocinations all come to naught, my famous insight into character proved utter folly. The diaries were lying on the hearth ready to be burned, but she told me to hold on, to wait awhile."

Mary Chestnut's wishes were ignored, and yours might be too, but if you want to destroy your journal, this isn't as unusual as it sounds. You might tear up your writ-

Ritual: A Ritual for Destroying the Fears in Your Journal

Life coach Susan Spritz Myers suggests this powerful ritual if you want to symbolically destroy and overcome the fears expressed in your journal.

1. Go through your journal and identify the fears you've written down.

2. Copy each fear on a separate piece of paper. As you do so, restate each fear aloud as a positive affirmation. For example, if you've written "I'm afraid I'll never lose that ten pounds," say "I am at my ideal weight, I feel healthy and look wonderful."

3. Carefully burn the pages one by one, repeating aloud the positive affirmations. Collect the ashes.

4. Choose a location that is meaningful for you, such as a mountaintop, the Grand Canyon, the sea or lakeside, or even the site where you first experienced a particular fear, such as the playground of your elementary school or the local baseball field.

5. Scatter your ashes to the wind.

6. As your ashes disperse so do your fears.

ing to protect someone you love; or on a happier note, if your journal is a catalog of fears you've overcome, you might want to symbolically destroy those fears and release yourself from their grip.

One of those fears might be that practicing total honesty in your journal will disrupt your life, but put this concern aside. It's essential for you to be forthcoming so the journal-writing process can do its work. You need to explore your ideas without internal censors or social inhibitions. You can't worry about being polite or hurting anyone's feelings, and it's only through total honesty that you can face your emotions and learn to deal with them.

"No legacy is as rich as honesty."

—WILLIAM SHAKESPEARE, *ALL'S WELL THAT ENDS WELL*

In fact, if you don't tell the truth, if you aren't honest with yourself, you may not find the answer to your question, the solution to your problem, or the cause of your pain. Now, sometimes this honesty may be quite eye-opening. You may even read your journal entry the next day and wonder who wrote it. However, if you're truthful, you will know it came from your authentic self, from some essential part of yourself you're just getting to know. Ultimately, this knowledge is power so don't be afraid.

Don't be afraid of trying to write either, urges poet, teacher, and journal expert Natalie Goldberg. Ironically, Goldberg explains, the key to overcoming this fear is to continue writing, and to do it without editing. Editing goes against the grain of keeping a journal. Instead, let the words flow. Feel free to spell by approximation and punctuate by chance, and don't worry about length or style. In fact, don't make any judgments at all, just put pen to paper and go for it. You'll be amazed at what happens. Virginia Woolf was.

"I got out this diary and read . . . the rough and random style of it, often so ungrammatical, and crying for a word altered, afflicted me somewhat . . . And now I may add my little compliment to the effect that it has a slapdash and vigour and sometime hits an unexpected bull's eye."

When you keep a journal, the very act of writing helps you hit your target. It puts you in control, gives physical form to your thoughts, and liberates your dreams. Journal writing allows you to channel your self-talk, translate misunderstood feelings, and mold the person you want to be. China Galland, author of *The Bond Between Women, A Journey to Fierce Compassion,* and founder and director of the Images of Divinity Research Project, says it is a way to discover the divine energy in yourself and move toward fulfillment as a human being—all that from the simple act of putting pen to paper. But with that pen and paper you are exhuming your past. You are projecting your future and charting your spirituality. You are honoring your experience and giving it worth.

Part of honoring your experience is respecting the paradox of journal writing. While it's true that your journal is a safe place where you can cover any topic and not worry about the world pointing fingers, you may end up pointing a finger at yourself. You may learn things in your journal that make you want to grow and change; this means your inner journey is progressing.

Exercise: A Breathing Exercise

In preparation for your journal-writing journey, try this simple breathing exercise, which is designed to create a sense of balance and focus that will help you write.

1. Choose a comfortable chair near a good light. For this first time, use a paper and pen. Physically clear the space so you have enough room to write. Now sit down and close your eyes.

2. Breathe rhythmically. Inhale through your nose and count slowly to four. Now exhale through your nose counting slowly to four. Repeat this breathing pattern three times.

3. Next, inhale through your nose and exhale through your mouth. Repeat three times.

4. Now inhale through your mouth and exhale through your nose. Repeat three times.

5. Finally, inhale through your mouth and exhale through your mouth three times.

6. Place a common object in front of you, something three-dimensional. This might be a flower, a candle, a piece of candy, anything with tactile qualities, smell, and color. Give yourself five minutes to describe it, but don't limit yourself to the object's physical qualities. Instead, think about the first time you encountered this item. What are your memories? Where were you? What was the temperature? Was the sun out? Were you alone? How old were you? What did you do with the object that first time? What else was happening around you? What did the day smell like? Were you wearing summer or winter clothes? Continue asking yourself similar questions.

Try the same exercise with a photograph of yourself or a loved one or choose a person to "talk to." Your mind will reward you with mountains of details that will help you uncover how you felt at the time.

This technique also will help you make mental connections. It will limber up your writing muscles and allow you to concentrate so you can begin your journey.

Responsibility

As you write each journal entry, you progress in taking responsibility for yourself. In so doing, you empower yourself to make a meaningful change. This is true regardless of why you keep a journal. No matter what your reason, you are taking responsibility for an area of your life and moving it forward just by writing about it.

And you can write about anything. No topic is taboo. In fact, it may be comforting to realize that people have poured out their feelings on similar subjects century after century. Chapter 3 will help when you're ready to select your specific topic. For now, it may be intriguing to see what others have written on various popular themes, as in the following journal entries.

ON THE AGING PROCESS:

"This period in my life seems to me very fine . . . my darling boys are growing more independent. I can already see the time when they will break loose from me . . . and I shall still be young enough for my own life."
—Kathe Kollwïtz, 1867–1945, graphic artist and sculptor
Written in April 1919

"Age is a desert of time . . . with little to do. So one has ample time to face everything one has had, been, done; gather them all in; the things that came from the outside, and . . . inside . . . time at last to make them truly ours."
—Florida Scott-Maxwell, Born 1883, playwright and Jungian psychologist, began keeping a journal in her seventies
Written in 1975

ON SELFISHNESS:

"How sick one gets of being good, how much I should respect myself if I could burst out and make everyone wretched for 24 hours; embody selfishness . . . the dolts praise one for being amiable! Just as if

one didn't avoid ruffling one's feathers as one avoids plum-pudding or any other indigestible compound!"

> —Alice James, 1848–1892, born New York City,
> sister of Henry James, reputed to be a frustrated writer
> Written on December 11, 1889

ON THE ENVIRONMENT:

"We find a bamboo root, three feet high. Very gnarled and sea-washed. Heavy. The beach is covered with them. They've made their way down streams, washed by rain into the sea, then swept by tides to the shore. Inside the house, tentacles of our root spread upward. We lean it against the table and admire its form."

> —Charlotte Painter, author of *Confession from the Malaga Madhouse*, a single mother
> Written in the 1950s

ON RELATIONSHIPS:

"Why isn't more said about the sensuousness between mother and baby? Men paint it and seem to assume it—women don't even mention it among themselves. Either it is completely taken for granted or it isn't considered at all."

> —Frances Karlen Santamaria, born in Cleveland, Ohio, a journalist since age fifteen, wrote about the events in her life
> Written on January 15, 1964

"I am so used to living not my own life but the life of Lyova and the children . . . It is sad that my emotional dependence on the man I love should have killed so much of my energy and ability; there was certainly once a great deal of energy in me. . . ."

> —Sophie Tolstoy, 1844–1919, long-suffering wife of the writer and gambler Leo Tolstoy (*War and Peace*), half his age, married at eighteen.
> Written in 1890

"Sometimes I am tempted to go to his house and pull on his door bell until the cord breaks. . . . I imagine myself lying down outside his door waiting for him to come out. I would like to fall at his feet . . . that would be madness—but I would like to throw myself into his arms and cry out, 'Why do you deny your love for me?'"

—George Sand, 1804–1876, admired writer,
acknowledged as one of the first "liberated women"
Written in November 1834, in Paris

ON WORKING:

"For many days, my brain worked with a dim and undetermined sense of unknown modes of being."

—William Wordsworth, 1770–1850, British Romantic poet,
author of *Tintern Abbey* and *Ode: Intimations on Immortality*

ON MEANING IN LIFE:

"One needs something to believe in, something for which one can have whole-hearted enthusiasm. One needs to feel that one's life has meaning, that one is needed in this world."

—Hannah Senesh, 1921–1944, born in Hungary, experienced
World War II, a Zionist pioneer who was tortured and executed
on November 7, 1944
Written in 1938 at age seventeen

What all of these entries have in common is the desire to answer the big questions of life:

+ Who am I?

+ Why am I here?

+ What's my true calling?

+ How can I know myself?

- Why am I the way I am?
- How can I create time and a life for myself?

Answers to questions like these don't come easy. At first your journal entries may pose more problems than they answer. This was certainly true for Maria Bashkirtseff, a young artist living in Europe in the 1800s who wrote the following shortly before her death at age twenty-four from tuberculosis:

"I have just been reading my journal . . . for 1875. . . . I find it full of vague aspirations toward some unknown goal. My evenings were spent in wild and despairing attempts to find some outlet for my powers. . . . What should I strive to become?"

Still, if you are persistent, enlightenment will dawn, as it did for British writer Joanna Field, whose journal, *A Life of One's Own,* served as an aid to self-analysis.

"I began to have an idea of my life, not as the slow shaping of achievement to fit my preconceived purposes, but as the gradual discovery and growth of a purpose which I did not know. . . . It will mean walking in a fog for a bit, but it's the only way. . . ."

The succeeding chapters of this book will help you use your journal to learn your purpose. Writing about your experiences exposes powerful patterns of behavior that can give you great personal insight and may lead to significant growth and change. This change will transform you and help you find your true calling. It will also acquaint you with your soul.

In fact, your journal is an excellent place to explore your soul and your spiritual life, bond with a Higher Power, request divine guidance, gain insight, and practice forgiveness, understanding, and acceptance. Incredibly, writing actually can help you cross the threshold of a brighter spiritual plane. It did for Kathe Kollwïtz, and this is the entry she made in her journal in September 1915:

"What can the goal of humanity be said to be? . . . The goal is the same as it is for the individual . . . first . . . happiness in love. . . . On a somewhat higher plane is the joy of self-development. Bringing all one's forces to maturity . . . the goal is to develop divinity, spirituality."

"Writing itself is one of the great, free human activities. There is scope for individuality and elation and discovery. In writing . . . the world remains always ready and deep, an inexhaustible environment, with the combined vividness of an actuality and flexibility of a dream. Working back and forth between experience and thought, writers have more than space and time can offer. They have the whole unexplored realm of human vision."

—WILLIAM STAFFORD, *WRITING THE AUSTRALIAN CRAWL*

The Stages of Spiritual Evolution

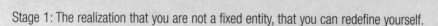

In his book *Spiritual Dimensions of Psychology,* teacher Hazrat Inayat Khan defined the stages of spiritual evolution as:

Stage 1: The realization that you are not a fixed entity, that you can redefine yourself.

Stage 2: Understanding that you can identify with the eternal, with something that doesn't die.

Stage 3: Knowing that you can move from personal consciousness to pure spirit.

Stage 4: Acknowledging that you are in a continual state of becoming, that you can give rebirth to yourself.

Stage 5: Knowing that you are more than "yourself," that you can discover your eternal archetype.

Stage 6: Expressing your eternal archetype through your personality.

Stage 7: Ultimately, you can come to understand the value of life, of what you have gained through living your life and what the Higher Power has gained through you. Discovering that a Higher Power can become human in you can help you discover your true potential for life.

You too can write about divinity and spirituality, and your explorations will lead you to your own stages of spiritual growth. Hildegard of Bingen, the eighty-one-year-old abbess of a convent in the Rhine Valley, wrote of this very experience in her journal more than six hundred years ago:

"I am life, complete unto itself, whole, sound, not needing stones to be sculpted, not needing branches to blossom nor rooted in human potency. Rather, all life has its root in me. . . . Some question Him. I wonder how then is it possible for God not to be at work? God is understanding."

The same understanding can be yours through the journal-writing process. This book will show you how. It will acquaint you with the art of journal writing, provide you with resources and techniques, stoke your creative fires, offer spiritual inspiration, and aid you in your personal transformation. All you have to do is begin. Of course, that is easier said than done, but you only need one word to start. Use any word that has meaning and power for you and know as you write this word that you are taking the first step toward writing your authentic self.

FOR MORE RESOURCES ON JOURNAL WRITING, READ:

Cameron, Julia. *The Artist's Way* (New York: Tarcher/Perigree, 1992).

Didion, Joan. "On Keeping a Notebook," in *Slouching Toward Bethlehem* (New York: Dell, 1968).

Edgerton, Franklin. *The Bhagavad Gita* (New York: Harper Torch Books, 1944).

Goldberg, Natalie. *Wild Mind—Living the Writer's Life* (New York: Bantam Books, 1990).

Goldberg, Natalie. *Writing Down the Bones—Freeing the Writer Within* (Boston: Shambhala Publications, 1986).

Khan, Hazrat Inayat. *A Meditation Theme for Each Day* (New Lebanon, N.Y.: Omega, 1982).

Monk of the Eastern Church. *Orthodox Spirituality* (Crestwood, N.Y.: St. Vladimar's Press, 1978).

Rimpoche, Sogyal. *The Tibetan Book of Living and Dying* (New York: Harper, 1994).

FOR MORE EXAMPLES OF JOURNALS, READ:

Bashkirtseff, Marie. *Marie Bashkirtseff: The Journal of a Young Artist,* trans. Mary J. Serrano (New York: E. P. Dutton, 1923).

Edel, Leon, ed. *The Diary of Alice James* (New York: Dodd, Mead, 1964).

Field, Joanna. *A Life of One's Own* (London: Penguin Books, 1955).

Frank, Anne. *Diary of a Young Girl* (New York: Doubleday & Co., 1952).

Kollwïtz, Kathe. *Diaries and Letters*, ed. Hans Kollwïtz (Berlin: Henry Regnery Co., 1955).

Nin, Anaïs. *The Diary of Anaïs Nin* (New York: Harcourt, Brace & World, 1966).

Painter, Charlotte. *Confessions from the Malaga Madhouse* (New York: Dial Press, 1971).

Sand, George. *Intimate Journal* (New York: John Day, 1929).

Santamaria, Frances Karlen. *Joshua: Firstborn* (New York: Dial Press, 1970).

Tolstoy, Sophie. *The Diary of Tolstoy's Wife 1860–1891*, trans. Alexander Werth (London: Victor Gollanz, Ltd., 1928).

Woolf, Virginia. *A Writer's Diary*, ed. Leonard Woolf (New York: Harcourt, Brace & World, 1954).

YOU MAY ALSO CONTACT:

China Galland at www.imagesofdivinity.org

Susan Spritz Myers
    Living From Your Heart
    P.O. Box 383
    Glencoe, IL 60022
    847-242-0351

2.

The Benefits of
Keeping a Journal

Keeping a journal has many benefits. It can aid you on the path of self-awareness, enlightenment, and growth by providing a secure forum in which to experiment. A journal also can help you balance perspective, release negative emotions, explore new options, and appreciate your accomplishments. In addition, writing regular journal entries is an excellent way to connect with your inner life. Why is this important? In the hustle and bustle of daily living it is increasingly difficult, sometimes impossible, to find quiet moments when you can reflect, yet these very moments are when insight, change, and growth occur. A journal encourages you to take time for reflection. So does reexamining what you've written.

If you've ever had the experience of discovering old photographs of yourself, you probably remember the moment of surprise, delight, or dismay as you thought "Look how I used to be!" You'll have the same reaction when you revisit old journal entries. In fact, your journal is a lot like a photo album, but instead of using a camera to record your life, you use a pen. Each entry preserves a particular experience and does it with tremendous power because layers of feelings and depths of emotions are captured in your own words. These words can help you develop clarity, truth, and trust.

Clarity

Clarity is the ability to see clearly and without obstruction. We all long for greater clarity in our lives, but it's often hard to see clearly in the flurry of daily activity. Your journal can help. Therapist and career counselor Barbara Sher uses life dreams to provide a powerful example of how this works. "Right now your dreams are as disorganized as a kid's closet," writes Sher. "In the back are boxes whose contents you can't remember anymore, and in front are all the dreams that were based on first-life illusions, now in terrific disarray ... but there's a new person in you ... that means all your dreams have to be reevaluated."

Your journal is the perfect place to undertake this evaluation. Start by identifying the most important things that ever happened to you from as far back as you can remember. Recall how these incidents felt, Sher suggests. List your percep-

---

Inspiration: Barbara Sher's "Support Your Local Genius Night"

To help clients make their dreams come true, teacher and career counselor Barbara Sher holds "idea parties" in which invitees gather to share strategies, establish goals, swap information, and provide mutual support. Examples of Sher's gatherings dubbed "Support Your Local Genius Night" include:

+ Brainstorming on financing a one-woman play

+ A mailing party to send out invitations to an art exhibit

+ A grant application party

+ Strategy sessions on escaping Corporate America

You can hold such a gathering to support yourself and others and to realize the dreams clarified in your journal.

tions, what you learned, and why a particular incident had a big impact on you. Now write the highlights of your life as others see them on another page in your journal.

You can guess at these opinions or you can interview people—your parents, siblings, teachers, and friends. Compare the two lists. Does anything surprise you? Those surprises are the first seeds of clarity your journal can provide.

For instance, you might discover that many childhood things that were important to you went unnoticed by your family. Friends may not realize that you were defined

An Interview with Ann Pardo on the Benefits of Journal Writing

Ann Pardo, a writer and licensed clinical professional counselor in Chicago, Illinois, uses journal writing in both her clinical practice and in her personal creative work. She has this to say about the benefits of the process:

Q: What are the benefits of journal writing?
A: Journal writing communicates what's deep inside you. It focuses issues. Writing entries is also validating because you can see something tangible right there in front of you.

Q: What does that validation do?
A: It allows you to try new things, to be excited about writing. I have one client who takes her laptop to . . . bookstores to write her journal entries. It makes her feel like part of things and brings energy to her writing and her life.

Q: What is the impact of journal writing on a personal level?
A: A journal gives you total control. You can take your entries as far as you want, you can expose yourself as much as you want to. Writing in a journal also has a nice kinesthetic quality to it, especially if you choose the right pen. In our fast-paced world, keeping a journal slows things down. It gets rid of extraneous stuff in life whether you use a pen or a computer, and that's a great thing.

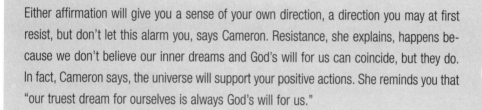

Inspiration: Affirmations from Julia Cameron to Help You Work on Your Life Dreams

Journal expert and teacher Julia Cameron writes that we must have the courage to admit our dreams and act on them. To make this pathway easier, she recommends the following affirmations:

+ "I know the things I know."

+ "I trust my own inner guide."

Either affirmation will give you a sense of your own direction, a direction you may at first resist, but don't let this alarm you, says Cameron. Resistance, she explains, happens because we don't believe our inner dreams and God's will for us can coincide, but they do. In fact, Cameron says, the universe will support your positive actions. She reminds you that "our truest dream for ourselves is always God's will for us."

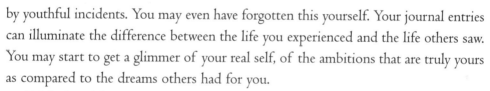

by youthful incidents. You may even have forgotten this yourself. Your journal entries can illuminate the difference between the life you experienced and the life others saw. You may start to get a glimmer of your real self, of the ambitions that are truly yours as compared to the dreams others had for you.

With this delineation in mind, write a history of your goals from as far back as you can remember. For example, maybe at age five you dreamed of having a puppy; at sixteen you wanted to be prom queen; at thirty to own your own business. Sher writes to be sure to include places you want to visit, things you want to do, and people you want to meet. Also note the things others have said about your aspirations and what you have told yourself, even the myths like "That's too hard," "I'm too old," or "It won't pay the rent."

"The idea is the means, but its breaking is the goal."

—HAZRAT INAYAT KHAN

Review what you've written, then go back and analyze what happened to each ambition. You may have simply outgrown some of them. Others may have been interrupted midstream. Maybe you were forced to conform; didn't take yourself seriously; were sidetracked by your success on another path; were living someone else's dream; felt insecure because of an earlier failure; or waited for an invitation that never came instead of asking for what you wanted.

As you examine these entries, ask yourself if your goals were given up for the same reasons. Study the patterns. Eliminate any goals you no longer want. As you write about this in your journal, your real dreams, the ones that represent your true calling, will become clear.

You can then use this clarity, states Sher, to design the action steps that will make your ambitions come true. More important, she concludes, you will see those dreams for what they really are—a message from your talents.

Discovering the connection between your dreams and talents is just one point of clarity your journal can provide. There are many others. Writing about issues that seem cloudy helps you visualize them and physically see connections. This in turn can lead to powerful realizations that might not have appeared had you not put them into words.

Truth

You must develop a taste for truth-telling if your journal is to be effective. Half truths won't work; neither will false assumptions. Only accuracy, sincerity, and integrity will do. After all, it takes honesty to reach understanding, and it is understanding that gives you the power to grow.

Part of your growth may mean acknowledging an eternal truth. Many religions and philosophies, including the Orthodox churches, Hasidic Judaism, Tibetan Buddhism, and others, share the concept of a truth that focuses on the positive and encourages you to live in harmony with your spiritual beliefs. This is why even the most mundane incidents can have vast spiritual implications. It is also why the attention you give to seemingly small details in your journal can help you learn the truth and, in that truth, says writer May Sarton, realize that "... there is

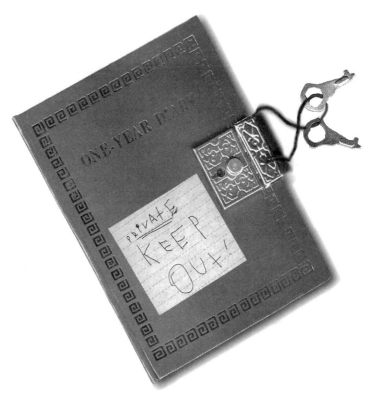

A young girl's first diary
from the journal collection of Olivia Lichens

nothing we do that is without meaning and nothing we suffer that does not hold the seed of creation in it."

Since everything you do has meaning, everything you write about can teach you something of the truth. This isn't to say you can't write about different versions of the truth. Often it may be helpful to do so. Just remember that in the end, you must write about your version, what *you* believe to be true. You also must not judge yourself if, once you've garnered more life experience, your perspective

"Before you can know the truth, you must learn to live a true life."
—HAZRAT INAYAT KHAN

on the truth changes. After all, the truth is based on where you are at a given point in time.

And if you're thinking that you don't have enough life experience to see the whole truth, your journal can help you work this through—but only if you trust it to do so.

Trust

As babies, we're small and helpless. We have little control over our environment, and our communication efforts are limited to wordless sounds. Thus we must trust our caregivers to nurture us and help us survive. Since our first feelings of confidence and acceptance are established at this time, we are all marked by these early experiences. Unfortunately, says research fellow and educator Maggie Scarf, even the best of caregivers may misinterpret our signals, and these misinterpretations can tarnish our sense of trust. Why does this happen?

Although Western culture emphasizes food, water, and shelter as the means of satisfying an infant's needs, anthropological studies show it's how these needs are met that's important. For instance, without affectionate physical contact, infant monkeys won't thrive even if their food and water dishes are full. The same is true for humans. Simply put, a little less food lovingly delivered is better than a banquet where the baby dines alone.

This sense of early deprivation, of violated trust, is a powerful memory of being in a vulnerable position and not trusting that it will be all right. It's why people often feel something was missing from their childhood, says Scarf, even though there were plenty of material goods to go around. Sometimes this feeling continues into adulthood.

"To become what you are, you must pass through a phase when you are nothing."
—ST. FRANCIS OF ASSISI, 1181–1226, FOUNDER OF THE FRANCISCAN ORDER
WHO RENOUNCED WEALTH TO FOLLOW CHRIST'S EXAMPLE

"Every child comes with the message that God is not yet discouraged of man."
—RABINDRANATH TAGORE, POET AND PLAYWRIGHT

Writing in your journal can give you an opportunity to reestablish the trust you may have lost as a child. Writer and researcher Carol S. Pearson, Ph.D., suggests that you start by creating a trust time line. Begin by thinking back to your childhood, as

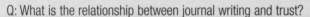

An Interview with Caroline Thomas, LCSW

Caroline Thomas, a licensed clinical social worker in private practice in the Midwest, offers these thoughts on building trust and other benefits of journal writing:

Q: What is the relationship between journal writing and trust?

A: Many of my clients, as youngsters, wrote journals, but Mom got hold of their journals and read them without permission. As a result, the whole issue of journal writing became associated with distrust. If you overcome this distrust, you can take advantage of the other benefits journal writing offers.

Q: Which are?

A: If you put your ruminating thoughts down on paper, move them out of your head, it's a cognitive shift. For instance, you might sleep better if you write before you go to bed. Also . . . if you keep a gratitude journal, it can help you be more optimistic about the future and show you that life's not so bad. For people who are really depressed or pessimistic, I have them write down the one hundred things they are most passionate about.

Q: What does that do?

A: It provides a sense of hope and optimism that there are things that provide pleasure and joy for you. It also starts the process of trusting yourself. Being truthful in your journal means knowing yourself, trusting who you are and who you can become.

> "Who is the wrong person to criticize? You."
> —IDRIES SHAH

far back as you can remember. Did you have everything you needed? As an adolescent, did you have a base of support so you could cast your net in the outside world? What was missing and why? Write it all down in your journal, then study the beginning of your trust time line carefully. If you can learn to understand your trust issues from the beginning, you can develop the skills to face the more daunting tasks of trusting your divine inheritance and trusting yourself.

Trusting yourself and having self-confidence are key to the journal-writing process. You must believe you have the power to communicate clearly with yourself through your journal and that you will do so regularly. You also must be willing to trust the paradox of journal writing so you can learn from your entries.

The paradox is this. While you can use your journal to write anything you want without fear of criticism, you actually may end up criticizing yourself in your entries. This often happens when you record disappointments and behavioral lapses, and make occasionally harsh self-judgments.

The trick to dealing with this, writes Julia Cameron, is to realize that you need

The Four Elements of Concentration

The following four steps to improve your concentration are based on Hazrat Inayat Khan's writings.

1. Observation/to lose one's self-consciousness

2. Contemplation

3. Meditation/communicating with the silent self

4. Realization, intuition, inspiration, and vision

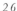

Atum O'Kane's Suggestions to Help You Develop a True Picture of Yourself

Nationally known Sufi teacher Atum O'Kane has several suggestions to help you uncover your true identity in your writing. First, picture yourself the way you want to be and write it. Remember to be kind to yourself. Value your need for beauty, ecstasy, glorification, and freedom. When you write about these desires, remember that they are real needs and attunements. Use these needs to uncover your life intention and evaluate whether this intention is being accomplished. Throughout this self-discovery process, experience yourself as a master. Then decide what quality you need to reach the master level and write about it.

both types of journal entries. You need nonjudgmental writing *and* self-criticism/self-analysis if you are to create a sense of balance and move ahead. Unfortunately, many journal writers forget to trust this fact. They don't realize that critical writing alone won't take them where they want to go. Neither will the nonjudgmental entries. Alone, each one is a skewed perspective; together they provide balance and balance in your writing offers the broadest possible range of benefits.

You can create this balance several ways. Some experts suggest separating different kinds of entries into different sections of your journal. Julia Cameron assigns basic tools each week to help you distinguish between the various emotional aspects of writing. Other instructors recommend starting with observation to lose your sense of self-consciousness and then working through different levels of concentration to aid in the writing process. Whatever their approach, each of these teachers expresses the need for balance in your entries.

Balance allows you to see both the positive and the negative in your writing. It helps you assess past issues fairly, evaluate present possibilities clearly, and have greater faith in the future. Developing balance doesn't mean you will experience instant transformation, but by trusting yourself and trusting the journal-writing process, you can begin to see a way of centering your life and creating the well-balanced person you want to be.

Greater Self-Knowledge

Your journal is a place where you can get to know yourself pretty well. Since we are the sum of our choices, whatever you write about can give you clues to who you are. It can reveal an area of concern in your life, record a standard you want to reach, acknowledge a success that bears repeating, or preserve a precious memory. It doesn't matter if you write about this topic in a judgmental or nonjudgmental way, as long as you remember that, over time, you are striving for balance. Balanced information, writes researcher Carol S. Pearson, leads to greater self-knowledge. With that in mind, your journal might include:

+ Self-criticism balanced by self-analysis

+ Disappointments balanced by achievements

+ Anger balanced by pleasure and satisfaction

+ Sadness balanced by joy

+ Restlessness and depression balanced by optimism and contentment

+ Hate balanced by love

+ Desire for revenge balanced by mercy, forgiveness, and reconciliation

+ Unfair treatment balanced by honesty and justice

+ Failure/having no luck balanced by victory

+ Being in the wrong place at the wrong time balanced by being in the right place at the right time

---

"I told Mother . . . to . . . write in my book . . . she wrote this to help me . . . 'make observations about our conversations and your own thoughts. . . . It helps you to express them and to understand your little self. . . . Remember, a diary should be an epitome of your life . . . a record of . . . thoughts and . . . actions.' "

—LOUISA MAY ALCOTT, AMERICAN AUTHOR, 1832–1888,

WROTE POPULAR NOVELS FOR YOUNG PEOPLE

This isn't to say you must seek out negative events and emotions on a daily basis, but by acknowledging them in your life, you will understand that these feelings are part of the human condition and out of their darkness comes light.

In addition, nothing can help you appreciate an emotion as much as experiencing its opposite. For example, writing about the joys of a partnership is all the more satisfying if you've been alone; writing about conflict resolution is more meaningful if you've experienced anger and frustration. Seeing such dichotomies laid out in your journal can be very illuminating. It was for Anne Frank, who wrote about it this way in her famous diary:

> "Sometimes, if I really compel the good Anne to take the stage for a quarter of an hour, she simply shrivels up as soon as she has to speak, and lets Anne number one take over, and before I realize it, she has disappeared. . . .

Besides self-knowledge, Anne Frank's diary also gave her a clearer perspective, as reflected in this journal entry written Wednesday, January 5, 1944:

> "This diary is of great value to me, because . . . on a good many pages I could certainly put 'past and done with.' "

You, too, may be able to write "past and done with" on certain episodes in your life as soon as your journal gives you perspective.

Perspective

Perspective is the lifelong process of arranging yourself in relation to your physical, emotional, and spiritual landscape, but there's a trick to it. Perspective changes constantly. Fortunately, your journal can help you keep track of your perspective wher-

---

"What fun it is to generalize in the privacy of a notebook . . . a great, delicious sweep in one direction . . . then with no trouble . . . an equally delicious sweep in the opposite direction. . . ."
—FLORIDA SCOTT-MAXWELL

"... Mr. Lane read a story ... how a rich girl told a poor girl not to look over the fence at the flowers and was cross to her because she was unhappy. The Father ... made the girls change clothes. The poor one was glad to do it and he told to her to keep them. But the rich one was very sad ... after that she was good to shabby girls."

—LOUISA MAY ALCOTT

ever it chooses to go. Your journal can also help you see why you might have different perspectives on the same situation and why these varying viewpoints are equally valid depending on where you are at the time.

Ultimately, your perspective determines whether you see a situation as an opportunity or a crisis. For instance, at different times permanent employment may mean economic security or being trapped; ending a relationship may set you free or make you feel abandoned; and so on. If you are stuck in one perspective, maybe it's because

Exercise in Perspective

The following exercise from Sufi teacher Atum O'Kane is designed to help you develop perspective. Try writing about it in your journal.

1. Imagine walking in the forest and seeing a snake. Your first reaction is fear and terror. You run as fast as you can to escape.

2. The next night you walk again, only this time you realize that what you thought was a snake is actually a rope. As you stroll away you feel relieved.

3. The third night out you see it again. It still looks like a snake but now you know it's a rope. You pick it up and use it to climb.

According to O'Kane, this exercise will help change your outlook or worldview. Simply replace "snake" with your issue or fear and then use these same steps to see anything in a different way. Write about these new perspectives in your journal.

you are invested in a particular point of view. Your journal can help you see this so that you can make a change, if necessary.

Your journal is also a good place to explore common perspectives and to consider some alternatives, such as these suggested by Carol S. Pearson:

Common Perspective: Being born to the "wrong" parents.
Alternate Perspectives: You "choose" your parents to complete unfinished spiritual business; to offer your soul a challenge; to gain maturity by being exposed to people you would not otherwise know; to practice forgiveness.

Common Perspective: Being in the wrong relationship. Alternate Perspectives: It was a misjudgment due to inexperience; you both changed; you discovered a lot about yourself; this experience is good training for future relationships; you learned forgiveness.

Common Perspective: Being born the wrong color, gender, or body type. Alternate Perspectives: Don't judge yourself by others; we're all better off than some people, worse off than others; it's who you are inside that counts; beauty is an individual assessment.

Remember, your perspective is what you know to be true at a given point in time, and it is valid until you decide to change it. Your journal can help you decide when this change should take place. By tracking your thoughts and observations, providing clarity about new truths and old ideas, your journal is a divining rod that not only

"When I was a kid seeing women on TV and in the movies who weren't beautiful but were funny, it made me understand that I didn't have to be beautiful, I could be me and I knew I was funny."
—WHOOPI GOLDBERG, ACTRESS, COMEDIENNE, AS TOLD TO THE ACTORS STUDIO

finds perspective but helps you find your way. Unfortunately, the way is not without its challenges, but your journal can help you there too.

Enhanced Problem-Solving Abilities

Some of the problems you face are personal. You may be in a high-stress job or concerned about your relationships. Other problems are more universal. You might worry

"Achievement gives great power, detachment gives greater power."

—HAZRAT INAYAT KHAN

> "Millions of boys face these problems and solve them in one way or another. They live, as Captain Ahab says, with half of their heart and only one of their lungs and the world is worse off for it. Now and again, however, an individual is called upon to lift his individual patienthood to the level of a universal one and try to solve for all what he could not solve for himself alone."
>
> —ERIK ERIKSON, GERMAN AMERICAN PSYCHOANALYST AND AUTHOR OF *YOUNG MAN LUTHER*

about humankind, ecology, world rights, justice, and peace. Whatever problem you're trying to solve, keeping a journal can help.

Your journal can start the problem-solving process by helping you identify the issue. Barbara Sher says this might take the form of an observation, a question, or an emotional reaction to a situation. Perhaps you identify the problem through a whole series of vague journal entries in which you finally see a pattern. You can even use a wish list to help you figure out what's going on.

Once you identify the problem, you can speculate on ways to solve it. One method for evaluating solutions is to write about most desired, least desired, and break-even outcomes. Next, consider what it would take to make each of these solutions come about. Use your writing to brainstorm, to plot different scenarios, and, if necessary, to temper your emotions so you can see the answers more clearly.

When you figure it all out, write an action plan. Be sure that your plan includes contingencies in case the situation changes or better options come along. Your journal can help you keep track of your progress. It can also provide you with a measure of comfort because even if your plans go awry, your entries are bound to show increased self-knowledge, a more thoughtful perspective, and a new way of connecting to yourself, others, and the world.

> "We have to believe that every person counts, counts as a creative force that can move mountains."
>
> —MAY SARTON

> "Writing a journal can be a form of prayer. . . . Look for passages that move you, inspire you, find wisdom rekindled. . . . It is a gift from outside ourselves."
>
> —CHINA GALLAND

Personal Growth, Wisdom, and Maturity

Whether you use your journal to solve a personal problem or to come to terms with a global situation, it's bound to impact your life in a positive way. In fact, your journal can be a key to improvement on many levels. Sometimes this growth is exhilarating and highly progressive. Other times it's slow going, painful, or startling. But never fear. Even the most reluctant realizations can lead to wisdom, maturity, and a better comprehension of the universe if you let them.

Ritual: Christina Baldwin's Stages of Silence for Writing in a Journal

1. The quest for wisdom is inspired by silence. Your journal creates form, story, and meaning from this silence.

2. Begin with a ritual of preparation. Turn off the phone, light a candle, or say a prayer. Try to use the same location for this quiet preparation.

3. State your intention out loud.

4. Focus and calm your mind with deep breathing, a phrase, or mantra.

5. Allow a profound silence to sweep over you. Quietly receive emotions, memories, and spiritual connections.

6. Return gently to your surroundings. Write in your journal.

Adapted from *One to One: Self-Understanding Through Journal Writing.*

Why does this happen? Author China Galland says it's because journal writing puts your psyche on notice that you want to be in dialogue. This invites a response and your journal is the container where that response can grow. To accomplish this growth, examine your life story with curiosity, wonder, and respect. Don't approach it as a broken vessel that needs to be fixed. Instead, says Galland, remember that previous experience is not necessary for journal-writing success, but boldness is. And it is boldness that forges the powerful link between what you think and what you write, between who you are and whom you ultimately become.

TO LEARN MORE ABOUT THE BENEFITS OF JOURNAL WRITING, READ:

Didion, Joan. *The White Album* (New York: Penguin, 1972).

Duerk, Judith. *Circle of Stones—Woman's Journey unto Herself* (Philadelphia: Innisfree Press, 1989).

Myss, Caroline. *Anatomy of the Spirit: The Seven Stages of Power and Healing* (New York: Random House, 1996).

Sand, George. *Intimate Journal* (New York: John Day, 1929).

Sexton, Anne. *A Self-Portrait in Letters* (Boston: Houghton Mifflin, 1977).

Tagore, Rabindranath. *Collected Poems and Plays* (New York: Macmillan, 1913).

YOU MAY ALSO VISIT THE FOLLOWING WEB SITE:

"Reasons for Journaling"
http://207.158.243.119/html/reasons.html

YOU MAY ALSO CONTACT:

Caroline Thomas, LCSW
Partners for Change
55 E. Washington
Chicago, IL 60602

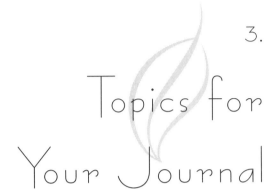

3.

Topics for Your Journal

Your journal allows you to study, sample, and sift through any topic. In fact, anything you care enough to write about is a good subject for your journal entries. You can focus on just one thing or, over time, cover a range of issues. You can even write about something different every day. Your entries can go into great depth or you can use your own private shorthand. You can organize everything in a single notebook or designate separate places for different subjects. It's your decision, but how do you choose what that first subject is going to be?

In the following pages we will examine some popular motifs and explore how you might individualize these in your journal. Offered are examples, resources, and ways to support you in your quest to find a topic that is meaningful for you. A good place to start is by asking yourself some of the following questions. Is there a long-held dream you're ready to begin? A need to communicate to future generations? A process or relationship you're trying to understand? The need to preserve a place or era? A specific goal you're trying to evaluate or spiritual issues you are exploring? Or do you just need an oasis in your life, a secure, private place where you can be you?

In addition to these personal subjects, you can also consider universal topics. Although these are as unique and varied as the people who write them, popular themes include: daily events; relating to nature; wellness and illness; family history;

> "The art of being happy lies in the power of extracting happiness from common things."
> —HENRY WARD BEECHER, 1813–1887, AMERICAN PROTESTANT CLERGYMAN,
> EDITOR, AND ABOLITIONIST LEADER

love; art and creativity; changing your avocation into a vocation; spirituality; money and material concerns; and your career. If you've never kept a journal before, you might want to begin with the first of these, the log of daily events.

The Daily Log

The daily log is exactly what it sounds like: a record of the incidents in your life that you consider meaningful or noteworthy. At first the log might appear to be a laundry list of random events. But seen over time, the daily log shows you how one experience leads to another, how a multitude of small elements can create a beautiful mosaic.

Ruth Larson Carlson who lived from 1898 to 1972, is not famous, but through her daily log, which her family agreed to share, she lives on. A Wisconsin farm woman, Ruth kept a journal for years recording: the weather; essential parts of farm life; seed, fertilizer, and basic staple prices; crop yields; milk checks; illnesses of family members both human and bovine; their recoveries; births; and deaths. Ruth's simple record of deaths led to deeper reflections, which brought a spiritual dimension to her writing and made her log the precious, insightful document handed down in her family. Some samples of these entries are:

"He's filled with cancer, as though it was the amount of cancer, as if it was only a little cancer, it wasn't so bad . . . Her husband died—eight children still at home—what will she do—I sure do

> "My flowers make me so happy, I have to keep my son Roy
> away from them with his lawnmower."
> —RUTH LARSON CARLSON, WRITTEN IN 1957

appreciate Dave, my husband. Sometimes you wish they'd go away for the whole day, but then you think what it would be like without them. Dave's a good man, loves the children, a nice sense of humor, not just for low sex jokes and loves to dance when he gets the chance, with me!"

Ruth's writing seems deceptively simple, but it's not. These straightforward entries led Ruth Larson Carlson to deep observations of her place in the world and her relationships with others. While it's true that her entries may seem unstudied, this is exactly why they are so powerful. The honesty and directness of her journal provides meaningful insight into this woman and her life. It allows Ruth to live on, not only for her family but for us.

Ruth's entries are also proof that the daily log is a rich place to begin, especially if you're concerned that your writing will lack depth or if you fear you have nothing to say. Her journal can teach you otherwise.

The Gardener's Journal/ Writing About Nature

Nature has been an inspiration for many writers, including teacher China Galland, author of *Longing for Darkness: Tara and the Black Madonna*, who addresses this topic with her students. "I first began writing a journal at the Grand Canyon. I was sitting by the water, painting and drawing, being inspired by the natural world; the soft colors are remarkable,

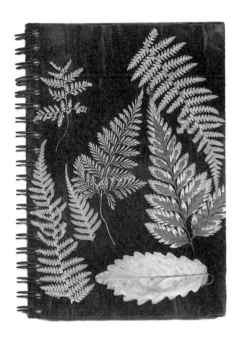
A gardener's journal
from the journal collection of the author

beautiful. My background is the wilderness, so I often have my students draw life as a river or I have them use a trail. Any natural image. It's a nonverbal exercise to find curves, bends, breaks, and then label them for writing or drawing."

Whether you admire a canyon in full summer leaf, create a magnificent garden, or simply want to understand why your houseplants don't thrive under your ministrations, writing about nature is a powerful way to connect with the earth and its life force. Gardening, raising crops, houseplants, or animals, and being attuned to the primal rhythms of the seasons are ways to experience the creation process. Writing about these experiences is reassuring because you can soothe yourself with the knowledge that everything in life ebbs and flows.

Galland notes that for many journal writers, nature and its cycles are the most convincing evidence that a Higher Power exists. As a result, nature entries can be a source of comfort and understanding. They can show you that in the greater scheme of things, your problems actually may be quite small.

By the same token, you as an individual are not small at all if you remember your connection with the natural world. Recording your observations of this world fuses the power of nature with the force of writing and spiritual energy. This potent combination produces entries that can spur significant memories, as revealed in these anonymous words from a fifteenth-century novitiate, written at age fourteen: "The roses bloomed, I yearn for my mother, the scent is her memory."

The nature journal can also help you understand the place of beauty in your life and

---

"Happiness is knowing a flower will grow where you've planted a seed."
—WRITTEN BY AN AMERICAN FARM WOMAN IN 1754

---

how a lack of beauty impacts your emotional well-being. This anonymous contemporary nature journalist observed of a friend: "Her house is like a graveyard for flowers. That must mean something." Whatever your entries mean, this type of writing will not only provide insights into Mother Earth's nature, but into your own.

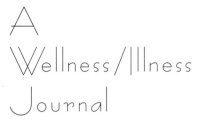

A Wellness/Illness Journal

Your journal can be a powerful healing tool to achieve wellness, understand illness, and promote recovery. It can aid you in putting spiritual flesh and bones on medical procedures that are all too often a frightening experience. How does this work? As you write, you will discover that you are not defined by your disease. Your journal entries support this realization because they allow you to distinguish between your ill self and your well self, between your eternal self and your external being. This distinction allows you to maintain your identity, marshal your positive resources, and focus on healing. In fact, many cancer patients insist that keeping a wellness/illness journal not only helped them track their progress, it helped save their lives.

This happens because cancer and other diseases are pivotal moments in life. Writing about these moments can transform your journal from a record of doctor's appointments, procedures, and bills, to a place of intense self-analysis, heartfelt emotion, and healthy support.

Your journal is also an excellent place to speculate on the meaning of life and the universality of your health experience. In addition, many people find that writing about illness and recovery brings them to greater spirituality, particularly as they learn the lessons taught by sickness and discover answers to the questions they ask. The progression from a wellness/illness journal that records the basic facts of the situation to one that provides healing for the soul often happens in a predictable sequence, say Carl, Matthew, and Stephanie Simonton, and James Creighton, a

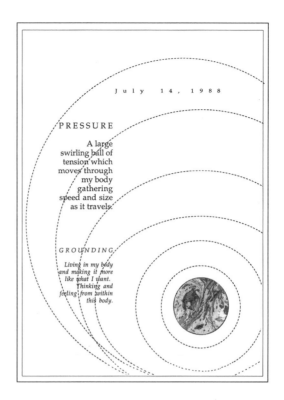

A page from a wellness journal
from the journal collection of the author

Creating Affirmation Pages for the Wellness/Illness Journal

To appreciate your wellness or help you recover from illness, visualize a fit, healthy, energetic you. Describe this image in positive, affirming words, such as "My body is healthy and zings with energy" or "I sleep deeply and well." Be aware that you may have to work through some fears, doubts, or your shadow self before you can write these positive statements in a convincing way, but that's okay. Facing and overcoming negativity or worst-case scenarios is key to the healing process.

medical doctor who helped the Simonton family cope with cancer. It is a sequence you may find helpful.

First, use your entries to assess your current state of health, including diet, exercise, and any information about the disease or genetics that apply to your situation. Next, write about any decisions you've made to change your health habits, especially the conflicts you feel and whether you've made peace with your hereditary issues. Use your journal to track your progress. No matter how your actions turn out, congratulate yourself for taking charge of the situation. You can also use your entries to talk to your body and to let your body talk back to you. One way to approach this in a journal entry is to ask yourself two questions. First, if your body could write you a letter, what would it say? Second, how would you respond?

Dialoguing with your body is a powerful use of your writing. So is dialoguing with your circumstances and writing about the impact of your health on loved ones. This makes your journal an effective coping mechanism. You may find yourself actively pursuing pathways that give you joy, peace of mind, and a sense of fulfillment. You might write about positive images associated with spirituality and health; analyze dreams for use in the healing process; document your experiences with a support group; or collect a list of jokes because studies show that extended periods of hearty laughter contributes to healing and deep, peaceful sleep.

The wellness/illness journal provides peace in another way too, because it helps you come to terms with your medical choices. It can aid you in preparations for the future, in exploring plans or legacies for loved ones, and in celebrating your passage to a new stage of life.

Whether that passage is a full recovery from illness or a peaceful, enlightened acceptance of a reduced level of health, it may seem like the logical ending point for your wellness/illness journal, but it's really only the beginning. Your experience and how you feel about it will become an integral part of who you are. Your journal can show you if you feel disempowered; it also can reveal renewed energy, better relationships, deepened spirituality, and an enhanced awareness of the beauty of life, regardless of how long that life may be.

Writing About Your Family History

Your family tree can yield an enormous harvest. Not only will it teach you about your ancestors, it will give you insight into your current family dynamics. As a result, you will have a clearer sense of where you are from, who you are, and what you have learned.

For most of us, the family is where we learned a particular set of rules, rules that came with certain expectations. If you spent your life with people of a similar race, economic, or social class, you may have assumed the same rules applied to everyone. Then, through life experience, you discovered that other people have different values, philosophies, and spiritual orientations. You were suddenly free to incorporate these examples or disregard them. For many journal writers, and perhaps for you, this crossroads is where your family history really begins.

If this is your starting point, your journal can help you determine if the old patterns are still a tried and true way of living your life or if some changes are required. Perhaps you wonder if there's a lesson in your family history that you can use to im-

Identifying Childhood Messages

This exercise is designed to help you identify some messages from childhood and see if they are still serving you well as an adult. Begin by closing your eyes and letting your mind drift back in time. Recall ten statements made to you in your youth and write them down.

You'll be surprised how many you remember. Were you told children should be seen and not heard? That you were too young to understand? Or did the dialogue go like this: "I wouldn't do that if I were you." "You'll never get it right. I'll do it for you." "You should be ashamed." "Don't do it, you'll get hurt." "Try it, you might like it." "Call me if you need me and I'll come get you, no questions asked." "You can do anything." "I'm proud of you." "I love you no matter what."

These messages are not necessarily good or bad. Still, they bear reexamination. After you take a close look, ask yourself if it's time to make a change, then write about your response in your journal.

prove relationships with your parents, spouse, or children, or if there are some skeletons you can clean out of your closet. Or maybe you just want to preserve memories for posterity. It really doesn't matter because these are all excellent reasons to start a family journal.

So is examining your family's impact on your behavior. We are all strongly influenced by our upbringing, states research fellow Maggie Scarf, and to some extent we are a reflection of our parents. As a result of this powerful influence, you might find yourself repeating certain ideas or work and relationship patterns in an effort to duplicate or change the way your earlier needs were met. If left unexamined, these patterns keep reasserting themselves generation after generation.

By starting with a chronicle of daily events and incidents, you can examine the

"If we learn how to forgive ourselves, to forgive others and to live with thanksgiving,
we need not seek happiness. It will seek us."

—ANONYMOUS, FROM THE FOURTEENTH CENTURY

patterns surfacing in your behavior and compare them to the rest of your family. You can base this comparison on your observations, recollections, and interviews with family members. You can also use your journal to practice family conversations you are not ready to have; to communicate with the departed; to plan ways to settle arguments; to confront someone who has hurt you; to apologize; ask for forgiveness; or express your love. Ultimately, this practice gives you the chance to achieve an intimacy and self-knowledge that might never be possible without the written page. It also gives you the opportunity to understand who you are within the family structure.

Another way to understand your family structure is to use your journal to study genealogy. Often people begin writing about their family's past when they reach mid-

Interviewing Relatives for Your Family History

You can use your journal to interview relatives for a family history. To help you create accurate entries, try asking these questions:

+ What is your full name?

+ What are the full names of your parents, siblings, in-laws, children, grandchildren, and great-grandchildren?

+ When and where were you born? When and where were your parents, siblings, and children born?

+ When, where, and how did your parents meet? You and your mate?

+ Describe your parents' education and occupations. Do the same for siblings, children, and yourself.

+ Are your parents and siblings still alive? Where do they live?

+ Do your parents have any brothers and sisters? Are they alive? Where?

+ Have you or your parents been married more than once? To whom? Are there children from these other unions?

dle age, states writer/genealogy researcher Lisa Ray Clewer. The average amateur genealogist is a man or woman forty to sixty years old; fifty-two is the median age. These demographics are not a surprise. Midlife is often a period of intense self-examination. You look at where you've been, where you are, and where you're going. You wonder if there's some clue in what others did with their lives. In addition, you are facing the loss of parents and older relatives who hold valuable information. Writing about your genealogy helps you preserve these resources, and often there are surprises in store.

One woman could never understand her family's negative attitude toward pregnancies. She chalked it up to superstition but then, while researching her genealogy, discovered that many of her relatives had children with cleft palates. This was cause for great shame and grief in her family's small Chinese village because the handi-

Questions for Use in In-Depth Interviews

In addition to mapping out the more factual aspects of your family tree, you can ask questions directed at discovering who family members really are. To do this, ask your relatives the following:

- ◆ How do you describe yourself?

- ◆ What special talents or hobbies do you have?

- ◆ What do you consider your greatest achievement?

- ◆ What are your professional and personal goals?

- ◆ What are your most important successes and failures?

- ◆ Has a particular person influenced your life?

- ◆ Where have you traveled and how did this affect you?

- ◆ What do you value most in life?

- ◆ Are there any family stories you want to pass on?

capped children had to be hidden and no one would marry into her clan. Eventually, this discovery led the woman to become an obstetrician. She wanted to use science to show her family that birth was nothing to fear and to create a greater acceptance of physical deformities.

Writing about genealogy can help you eliminate fear. It can also help you gain self-knowledge and see your family in a different light. As you ask questions and explore your past, you will gain a greater understanding of who you are, a broader picture of where you are from, and greater insight into where you and your family are going. With your journal as a guide, this can be a journey not only of genealogy but of enlightenment, truth, compassion, and love.

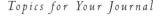

Love

Just as love is one of the most powerful of all human experiences, it is also a powerful topic for your journal—and it can be a challenge to write about. Why? When things are going well, says analyst Robert A. Johnson, people tend to write less or to write descriptions that are too one-sided to supply much insight. By contrast, when things get difficult, people may find themselves writing a lot, but that same one-sidedness might still apply. For this reason you might want to consider a more helpful approach. Instead of using your journal to figure out your lover, use it to learn about yourself in love.

Start by making a list of what you want to know. You might ask if you are truly yourself with this person or if you've had to make uncomfortable compromises; if you are equals and the relationship is one of balanced give and take; or if you have the same value systems. Look at both the positive and negative aspects of your behavior. Do you recognize any cycles?

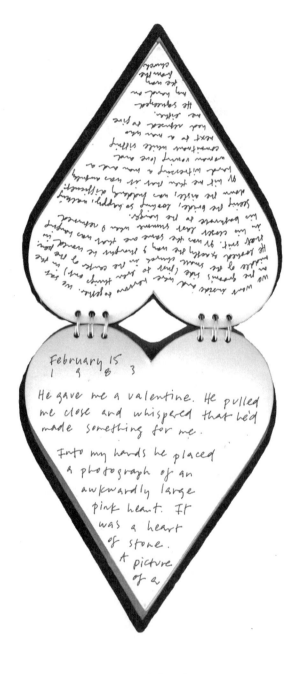

A journal about love
From the journal collection of the author

Robert Browning, the great Victorian poet, began to keep a journal upon meeting and falling in love with his soul mate and fellow poet, Elizabeth Barrett. His journal, devoted to his passionate feelings for Elizabeth, recorded the date of each visit and the length of time they spent together. Theirs was a relationship that overcame numerous obstacles, including Elizabeth's frail health, her dependency on her possessive father, and the varying successes of their careers. In his journal, Browning wrote: "Love was to feel you in my very heart and hold you there forever through all chance and earthy changes."

By using your entries to broaden your consciousness and develop your individuality, you enhance your ability to love and be loved. You also learn that love starts within, and this is where your growth and transformation begin. Often you see the first signs of this in your journal as you make note of your increased emotional gen-

An Exercise to Help You Write About Yourself in Love

Sometimes it's difficult to put an intensely emotional experience like love into words, especially if you're not sure that it's really love you're feeling or if you're in turmoil because things aren't going well. The following exercise uses a nonverbal technique to help you visualize yourself in love. This may make it easier to translate your feelings into words for your journal.

1. Imagine an ideal landscape, then draw it.

2. Now analyze your picture. Many psychologists say the left side is the past, the right side is the future. If you move from left to right, you see yourself in the future. If you move from right to left, something in the past may be holding you back.

3. Look at the colors you've used and where you placed yourself in the picture. Look at where or if you drew your lover. What is his or her spatial relationship to you? What does this say about your relationship?

4. Is your picture what you want to see? If so, you're on the right track. If not, articulate your challenges, fears, and concerns so you can create a better picture.

> "One of the beautiful things about the structure of the unconscious in human personality is that when it is time for growth, the old ways, the old habits pave the way and welcome the new. They seem to persecute the new growth at every point, but who knows, perhaps this is the correct way to bring a new consciousness to birth. . . . Often when new growth occurs, the most dreadful things seem to happen, but one sees that they were exactly what was required."
> —ROBERT A. JOHNSON

erosity, renewed self-confidence, and the sheer physical vitality and spiritual joy that come from love, this unique human experience.

Another unique human experience you may wish to write about is your love for your children. It is a powerful way of expressing dreams and excitement, fears and in-securities as you rearrange your life to take on a parental role. If you're new at par-enthood, your journal is an excellent place to tackle any concerns you feel as you change your schedule to make room for a child in your life, examine any stereotypes you may hold about being a parent, and write about what your child has taught you about yourself.

Your journal can also help you celebrate your child's talents, accept his weak points, and illuminate strong points you might otherwise not see. In addition, writ-ing can be a big help when you are angry. You can vent your frustrations on your jour-nal pages instead of on your child. A journal is a parental aid in another way, too, because your entries can reflect patterns in your child's behavior that you're too close to observe. Lecturer and physician M. Esther Harding said these can provide you with observations, perceptions, and a chronology you can use to track changes in your child's actions, attitudes, and health. In this way, your entries become a reference that not only helps you guide your child but helps you guide yourself as a parent. This makes your journal a tremendously valuable resource that no pile of photo albums or videotapes can ever replace.

In fact, preserving irreplaceable moments is an excellent reason to begin the writ-ing process. Whether it's the first visit from the tooth fairy, high school graduation, or your child's birthday, your journal is a treasure box where these memories can live. In fact, birthdays can be an excellent topic all on their own.

Birthdays

Whether it's a means of measuring your own life milestones, passing important information down to your descendants, or creating a wonderful gift for your child, birthdays provide markers by which we measure and reflect on the years. The birthday journal is a very satisfying way to record the fleeting experiences of childhood and provide a record of developmental stages in your youngster's life. It's also a tender keepsake for you, the parent, and a way to reflect on the lessons you've learned from your child.

A birthday journal can be a long-term project that starts at birth or before, and is then presented to a child on her eighteenth birthday, the traditional start of adulthood. Another option is to give the birthday journal to your child as an annual gift. Either way, a good format is to write your entries as letters. This creates an instant connection and allows your personality to flow freely through your words.

Try writing once or twice a month for the first five years so you can capture all the highlights and changes that take place during this precious, all-too-brief stage. Be sure to include passages about your relationship, and don't hesitate to write entries that cover both the high and low points. Not only will this benefit your child, but it will give you some perspective since, at a later date, you may discover that what you thought were disasters were really enlightening, often amusing, moments of growth.

Another way to write about growth in the birthday journal is through a questionnaire you design that identifies specific aspects of your child's personality at a given time. The

Example of a Birthday Journal Entry

The following entry is from a birthday journal written by a mother to her two-year-old daughter.

"When I get you out of your bed in the morning, you greet me with 'Hi, I love you!' One morning when I came to you, we looked out the window together. 'It's raining,' you said. 'Yes,' I replied, 'the sun isn't shining today.' To which you said, 'I see the raindrops on the trees. They take a drink.' I am impressed by your growing ability to appreciate and make sense of the world."

questionnaire can cover favorite things, including food, colors, friends, songs, books, activities, clothes, and toys, as well as new travel, language, and social experiences. You can design this yourself or with the help of your child. You can also illustrate the birthday journal with favorite snapshots and pieces of your child's artwork created in response to your entries. This collaboration makes the birthday journal more meaningful for you both. It also helps communicate all the important experiences and events that form the core of your child's life and to illuminate the loving relationship you share.

Friendships

Friendships are a wonderful topic for your journal because writing about them helps you appreciate your key relationships and how they grow. In addition, entries about good friends can help if you're feeling lonely or isolated. All you have to do is open your journal to find people who love and support you and who are rooting for your success. In fact, your friends probably will make regular appearances in your writing. You might even want to include some of their letters among your entries.

Two hundred years ago, the inclusion of letters in journals was a common practice, and it may work for you today. Notes from friends can remind you of what you were doing and thinking, how the relationship was progressing, and who you were at the time. You can also write letters to friends directly in your journal pages. You might find this technique loosens up your style, making it less self-conscious than normal. If you're ever stuck writing journal entries, this is a good trick to remember—just pretend you're writing to a friend.

Fortunately, the best thing about writing to friends in your journal is that you don't have to pretend at all. In your entries you can be absolutely upfront about the most complex and heartfelt aspects of your relationships and develop a sense of gratitude for the precious individuals who people your pages and fill your life.

"The thread of our life would be dark, Heaven knows!
if it were not with friendship and love intertwin'd."
—THOMAS MOORE, PH.D., PSYCHOTHERAPIST AND WRITER, LIVED AS A MONK FOR TWELVE YEARS

> "The Eskimo has fifty-two names for snow because it is important to him;
> there ought to be as many for love."
>
> —MARGARET ATWOOD, CONTEMPORARY CANADIAN AUTHOR AND NOVELIST

Writing About a Specific Emotion

Emotions are the filter through which all experiences pass, and they are a rich, provocative topic for your journal entries. You can use your writing to examine a whole range of feelings associated with a particular situation, or you can study one emotion in depth, over time. The latter can be extremely useful if you're trying to develop a positive frame of mind.

For instance, in a joy journal you can write about things that make you happy. You can describe both the emotion and your physical reaction to happiness, whether it's a high-powered rush of adrenaline or the soft purr of contentment. If there comes a time when life isn't going so well, you can look through your joy journal to reaffirm

Some Words of Wisdom to Help You Cope with Anger

Following are some common words of wisdom about anger that may be helpful the next time you feel this intense emotion.

- ✦ Pick your battles.

- ✦ Direct your anger at the right person, in the right place, at the right time.

- ✦ Use your anger to explain the harm done.

- ✦ Don't use your anger to retaliate, use it to correct the situation.

- ✦ Anger should be in proportion to its cause.

- ✦ Don't displace your anger onto an innocent party.

- ✦ Terminate your anger when the situation is corrected or you receive an apology.

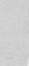

> "Happiness is not a state to arrive at, but a manner of traveling."
> —MARGARET LEE RUNBECK, BRITISH WRITER

your blessings and help you make it through the tough moments. A gratitude journal does something similar. Feeling thankful puts you in a state of grace. Writing about it helps you appreciate all the richness in your life, opens you to new abundance, and builds your sense of optimism and self-worth. This can be extremely helpful when you're faced with an occasional bout of the blues or if you feel depressed.

In fact, providing help is what keeping an emotional journal is all about. Because an emotional journal shows you very accurate patterns of responses related to very specific triggers and incidents, it is a useful tool. It can help you pinpoint negative feelings, reinforce positive ones, change behaviors, and cut through mental fog, even when you're dealing with an emotion as confusing as anger.

Anger often leaves people with their heads spinning, their adrenaline pumping, and nothing to show for it. Journal writing helps you name this emotion, find its source, and learn how to deal with it in a positive way. In journaling, says Dr. Sandra Thomas, founder of the Women's Anger Study, try to write while the anger is still fresh in your mind. Identify who or what triggered your feelings. Include the person's gender and status, then record your reaction. Were you aggressive? Accommodating but hating yourself for it? Victimized? Assertive?

After you describe your response, consider your physical sensations and reactions. Did you get a headache or stomachache? Eat chocolate? Cry? And what about your other emotions? Did you feel guilty, depressed, embarrassed, or have angry dreams? Finally, try to pick out the real anger trigger. With this information from your journal you can foresee anger incidents, be on the lookout for themes that set you off, and, if you choose, modify your behavior and then congratulate yourself on a job well done.

This last point is especially important. No matter what aspect of your emotional self you investigate, it's essential to pat yourself on the back for having the courage to face your feelings. By using your writing to celebrate these efforts, your journal becomes an honest barometer and a pathfinder, a friend that can help you avoid near drownings as you navigate life's sea of change.

The Visual Journal

The journal is essentially a written medium, but if you find putting words on a blank page intimidating, it might be easier to start with something visual as your topic. Since visuals speak more to the unconscious and intuitive part of you, the visual journal is an excellent way for nonwriters to begin. Pictures are inspiring, and ultimately written words will develop from the feelings that arise.

Eileen Kitzis, artist and director of the International Center of Photography/New York University Graduate Program in Photography, teaches classes that include "The Visual Diary," "The Healing Image," "Snapshots and the Retrieval of Memory," and "Storytelling." What these classes share is an equal emphasis on the visual and the verbal. "I strongly believe in the simultaneous workings of both these modes, otherwise known as left- and right-brain functioning," says Kitzis. "I believe that we are always experiencing life through what we see with our eyes and the words, language, and sounds going on in our heads. These two stimuli are truly interactive, like a Möbius strip. I honor both because they radically affect each other."

To work this way, select a blank book that is very special to you, one you enjoy having around. "It should be an object which you feel comfortable enough to bring into the bathtub or even spill coffee on. It should be kept with you at all times so that it is always there waiting to be paid attention to and receive," says Kitzis. She recommends keeping your journal next to your bed at night in case you wake up and want to write.

Once you've selected your journal, make a collection of two-dimensional objects. These should be things you encounter in your day-to-day life like a bus pass, theater tickets, or newspaper clippings. Kitzis says, "Any of the little scraps of life that attract you, stop you, and make you say 'Oh wow!' are suitable." Place them in your journal. In addition, record your dreams.

Now use the "oh wow!" collection and your dreams as a source of inspiration for your words. Start with automatic writing. Just string together your stream-of-consciousness thoughts; don't worry about whether your entries make literal sense. Eventually a specific topic, theme, or direction will emerge. It may even prove to be the inspiration for an art project.

Taking Notes on Your Dreams

To maximize your dream imagery and incorporate it effectively in your visual journal, try the following suggestions.

+ Immediately upon waking, write notes about your dream or use a tape recorder to capture your thoughts before you get out of bed.

+ Take notes throughout the day as you think about the dream.

+ Give your dream a title. Use the highlight of the dream to direct you and make the title an intuitive, emotional choice.

+ Note any dominant colors or forms in your dream and find a picture to illustrate them. You can also draw your own image. Remember, stick figures are just fine!

+ Create a private dictionary of symbols from your dreams and keep adding to it so you can distinguish patterns and better understand yourself.

You may also find a topic through other visual sources. Besides the "oh wow!" collection, look for images in magazines, newspapers, mail-order catalogs, rubber stamps, photo albums, and correspondence. Whatever you choose, there are only two things to keep in mind. First, don't select precious, one-of-a-kind imagery unless you're prepared to cut and paste it. Second, don't select images or objects that can't lie relatively flat on the page.

Now paste your pictures on the page. As you assemble them, be sure to leave room for other artwork and writing. When your visuals are in place, sit quietly in a comfortable position and let your body relax. Focus on breathing and imagine that with each inward breath you are filling your body with a golden light. Each time you breathe this light grows stronger and brighter, and your body becomes more deeply relaxed. When you feel calm and centered, slowly open your eyes and focus on the image you have selected.

Ask yourself these questions: What does this picture tell me about myself? Why do the colors or forms appeal to me? Why did I select this image? Connect the picture with

Creating a Treasure Map

Massachusetts-based organizational consultant Ingrid Bredenberg uses visuals to help students create a Treasure Map and inspire journal writing. These steps are from her class "LifeShaping: Designing Extraordinary Futures."

+ Start by visualizing your ideal day. In your mind's eye create an ideal home setting, work environment, or relationship. Be sure to include beauty, efficiency, and comfort when constructing your ideal. Select one area on which to focus.

+ Search through magazines for images and words that capture or represent the elements of your dreams. Turn your collection of pictures and words into a collage.

+ You may use a page of a blank book, a sheet of loose paper, or a photo album with sticky pages that allow you to construct your picture without glue. Each page of your visual journal can focus on a different area and represent a different goal.

+ Once you have your collage image, create and write down an affirmation to go with it. The affirmation should be something that empowers you to accept this possibility in your life. Bredenberg suggests, "This or something better now manifests with grace for the good of all." Revisit your pages regularly and meditate on the imagery. Observe and note what the process of constructing your Treasure Map has brought to you. Bredenberg believes that creating an image/word collage that embodies your desires, wishes, dreams, and goals is the best way to manifest what you want in your life.

something in your past, present, or future and write about it in your journal. Let the visual information liberate your words, then place those words anywhere you want—across the picture, around it, or underneath. When you finish writing, feel free to make your own drawing or decorate the page based on thoughts and feelings inspired by your entries.

And don't be surprised if these entries practically write themselves once you start working with visual topics. This happens because images often bypass your conscious, more judgmental mind to evoke raw feelings, recapture lost memories, and move you on a deeper level, a level where language pours out. The result can be cleansing and a great liberation for your creative self.

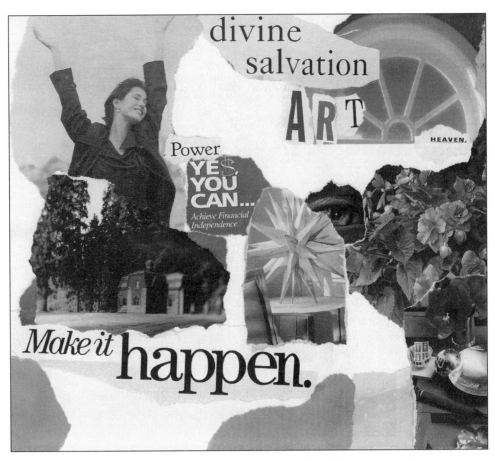

An artist's "treasure map" for manifesting prosperity and a full-time career making art

Writing About the Spiritual Journey

For centuries people have inquired about the meaning of life, what's beyond our physical, temporal world, and their place in the spiritual universe. While your initial entries on these matters might begin with a lot of thoughtful meandering and vague speculation, eventually your journal will get very specific in your quest for answers.

As you research various spiritual paths, you may try out different disciplines. You can choose from Buddha's thoughts on the meaning of life, the teachings of Muhammad, Job from the Bible, Hindu perceptions of the cosmology, ancient Egyptian spirituality, Native American beliefs, and many more. The spiritual journal is where you can explore your adherence to your chosen discipline and its effect on your life. As teacher China Galland says, your journal allows you to take note of where you find spiritual water, food, safety, and sustenance for your soul.

Money: Friend or Foe?

At the most basic level, a money journal is a record of incoming and outgoing cash, but if you look a little deeper, it's really something more. The money journal can re-

Creating Time and Space for Your Spiritual Practice

Sufi teacher Atum O'Kane suggests these steps to create a place for your spiritual practice. First find a private space. If necessary, turn off your phone or place a DO NOT DISTURB sign on your door. Try to make the time and place consistent. Native Americans, Tibetans, and Sufis believe there is a window between the ethereal world and the active world at 4:00 A.M. and say this is the best time for prayer and meditation. Books and teachings from your chosen discipline can guide you in this matter. Just remember that the practice itself is more important than the hour at which you do it.

Next, create a ritual for your practice using music, candles, incense, a special mat, or whatever properly sets the stage for you. Perform the spiritual practice. Don't expect immediate miracles, simply focus on being yourself within the practice.

If you get distracted start again or, if you like, find a teacher who has explored the practice you're undertaking. While your journeys will not be the same, sometimes a "map" in the form of an instructor is helpful.

flect patience and persistence as you watch your savings grow, a desire for instant grat-ification if you spend every cent you have, a sense of insecurity if you need to buy lavish gifts to impress your friends, or an emotional issue if you spend more money when you're depressed. When you use your journal to write about these patterns, it becomes a useful tool for identifying areas of potential growth and finding cycles of true abundance in your life—abundance that often has nothing to do with your bank account.

One way to discover these hidden messages is to write about your earliest money memories. Certified financial planner and bestselling author Suze Orman explains that these memories are the source of your money fears today. Recognizing these fears and giving them a name is one way to start down the road to financial freedom. Examples include "It's too expensive . . . we're broke" . . . "they're trying to rip us off" . . . "I would never spend money on that" . . . "It's their own fault they're poor" . . . "It's the bill collector! Tell him I'm not here!" . . . "I can't afford to make a donation! I've got to take care of myself first" . . . "Just use your credit card!" . . . "Buy it! You deserve it!" . . . "But it's on sale!"

Take a close look. Are these memories still influencing your life today? Use your money journal to explore this topic and see if these ideas are serving you well or if they're holding you back. You can also use your journal to set financial goals, to ex-plore changing circumstances and attitudes about money. What you learn may sur-prise you.

For instance, maybe you lost your job and this forced you to make some lifestyle adjustments. At first you weren't too happy about this, but then you notice that your journal reflects less stress because you have fewer *things* to take care of. In addition, you're spending more time with your children and spouse. Suddenly you have the free-dom to take a class, do volunteer work, or anything you want as you begin to experi-ence the joys of voluntary simplicity. This sets you on a new life course, and what's the end result? For the investment of a little time and thoughtfulness, your money journal pays big dividends in quality of life.

A Career Journal

Is your career everything you want it to be? Do you love what you do? Have you found your perfect calling? The career journal is an excellent place to explore these issues. It is especially useful if you've tired of your current profession, don't know

The Practical Power of the Financial Journal

Paula Dorion Gray, a Certified Financial Planner with Dorion Gray Financial Services Inc., Crystal Lake, Illinois, has this to say about the practical power of the financial journal:

Q: What is the practical value of keeping a money journal?
A: It's a good way to keep track of expenses. You can even put your detailed, monthly credit card bill in the journal as a record to see where you're spending money. Those with a tight cash flow can keep a notebook journal with them at all times and write down whatever they spend. This might sound tedious, but people need to be aware.

Q: How can you use a money journal on the income side?
A: Use your paycheck as a guide for a journal entry and use your journal to keep track of your 401K plan. Write it down so you can see how much you're saving. Most people have no idea how much money they have. Often they're surprised until they use a journal to track their expenses, income, and net worth.

Q: What does this do for the journalist psychologically?
A: Psychologically, it's good to see your money grow . . . It encourages us to do more saving . . . Tracking this in a journal builds our sense of security. I had a client, a young man, who started with nothing, but he began writing and keeping track and set aside $45,000. Now he has enough cash to pursue his acting career. He's mentally and financially ready to go. This gives him a sense of security and well-being. Physically seeing your thoughts and finances on paper helps people and it can help you.

what you want to do, or have put your creative self on hold. Just recognizing this in your journal is a step toward balance, and it might even inspire you to go a little further.

You might decide to pursue your creative dreams as a full-time vocation and your journal can help this come about. To use your journal this way, start by underlining any sentences that refer to work you'd like to do, writes therapist and career counselor Barbara Sher. After a month, go back and review these sections. Which idea pops up regularly?

Having found this idea, ask yourself what you can do to nurture it. Can you do research at the library or on the Internet? Take a class or talk with someone in your field of interest? Spend ten minutes each day focusing on your creative idea. If you lose enthusiasm, discard the idea and move on to something else. If, after a month, the idea still excites you and feels more like fun than work, you've found the focus for your creative plan. Now write a list of ways you can create time to make this plan come true.

While there's no question that it will take time, when you find the right idea,

An Exercise for Getting Over Creative Dry Spells

Everyone experiences creative dry spells. The following exercise inspired by author Linda Schierse Leonard can help.

1. Find a book of short affirmations or meditation quotes.

2. Sit quietly and center your breath.

3. Select an affirmation or quote for the day.

4. Read it several times.

5. Does it resonate with your life? Does it resonate with your work?

6. Write a few lines about the resonance this idea has with your life, then focus on your work.

7. By tapping into what inspires you, you can stop focusing on your dry spell and access your innate creative energy.

you'll know it. You will feel intrigued and excited; because you can hardly wait to see what each new day will bring as you move closer to your true calling and the realization of your life's work.

As you move into this work, your career journal can help you fine-tune your plan. It can show you if you're a specialist or a generalist, if you prefer to be part of a team or to work alone, or whether you like being in management. You can note the progress of individual assignments or training courses you undertake, discover your strong and weak points, ideas you need to develop, and when you're ready to move ahead. In addition, a journal can be especially helpful if you're thinking of forming a partnership because it can reveal patterns and allow you to anticipate certain eventualities. For instance, your entries may show you that both you and your partner have complementary strengths or that you both dislike dealing with money and you need some support in this area, and so forth.

Whatever the case, a career journal can help you see things more clearly. It provides a sense of clarity and truth that allows you to trust yourself, assess new risks, and feel secure on your chosen professional path.

Additional Options for Journal Topics

Additional subjects for your journal might include a travel journal to help you grow and integrate new experiences; a food or holiday celebration journal; a journal of movie or theater performances, a political journal; a current event journal; a journal of auditions; a fishing journal; an inspiration journal.

Other Options

The topics we've explored in this chapter are but a handful of the many you might consider for your journal. Ultimately, the choice is yours and no choice is wrong. No matter what you select, you will learn something important about the subject and yourself. Just making a selection will help you feel more decisive. It will focus your concentration, harness your energy, and give you insights to drive your life forward to the place you want to be and the person you want to become.

TO LEARN MORE ABOUT JOURNAL TOPICS READ SOME OF THESE RESOURCES:

Breathnach, Sarah Ban. *Simple Abundance: A Daybook of Comfort and Joy* (New York: Warner Books, 1995).

Cameron, Julia. *The Artist's Way* (New York: Tarcher/Perigee, 1992).

Campbell, Joseph. *The Hero with a Thousand Faces* (Princeton, NJ: Princeton University Press, 1949; reissued 1990).

Clewer, Lisa Ray. *How to Find Your Own Roots—A Guide to Tracing Your Family Genealogy and Making a Living History Album* (New York: The Works, 1977).

Ferguson, Marilyn. *The Aquarian Conspiracy* (New York: J. P. Tarcher, 1980).

Goldberg, Natalie. *Wild Mind—Living the Writer's Life* (New York: Bantam Books, 1990).

Harding, M. Esther. *The Way of All Women* (New York: Harper Colophon, 1970).

Harding, M. Esther. *Woman's Mysteries Ancient and Modern* (New York: Harper Colophon, 1971).

Herrigel, Eugene. *Zen and the Art of Archery* (New York: Vintage Books, 1971).

Johnson, Robert A. *HE Understanding Masculine and SHE Understanding Feminine Psychology* (New York: Perennial Library, 1986).

Koch, Kenneth. *Wishes, Lies, and Dreams* (New York: Vintage Books, 1970).

Leonard, Linda Schierse. *Witness to the Fire: Creativity and the Veil of Addiction* (Boston: Shambhala, 1989).

Orman, Suze. *The Nine Steps to Financial Freedom* (New York: Crown, 1997).

Pearson, Carol S. *Awakening the Heroes Within: 12 Archetypes to Help Us Find Ourselves and Transform Our World* (San Francisco: Harper San Francisco, 1991).

Pennebaker, James. *Opening Up: The Healing Power of Expressing Emotion* (New York: Guilford Press, 1997).

Pincus, Lily, and Christopher Dare. *Secrets in the Family* (New York: Pantheon Books, 1978).

Sandburg, Carl. *Always the Young Strangers* (New York: Harcourt, Brace & World, 1953).

Scarf, Maggie. *Intimate Partners* (New York: Random House, 1987).

Sher, Barbara. *It's Only Too Late If You Don't Start Now* (New York: Delacorte Press, 1998).

Sher, Barbara, with Anne Gottlieb. *Wishcraft* (New York: Ballantine Books, 1983).

Simonton, Carl, Matthew Simonton, Stephanie Simonton, and James Creighton, *Getting Well Again: A Step-by-Step, Self-Help Guide to Overcoming Cancer for Patients and Their Families* (J. P. Tarcher, 1978).

Stock, V. E., ed., *The Love Letters of Robert Browning and Elizabeth Barrett* (London: Century, 1987).

Treasure of Friendship, The, selected by Peter Seymour (Hallmark Edition, 1968).

ADDITIONAL RESOURCES:

Y-Me is a national support group for those facing the challenge of breast cancer. Members are taught to use wellness/illness journals and one of the first things they write about is "why me?" Y-Me can be reached at 1-800-221-2141. Many other support groups also use journal writing as a means to clarity, recovery, and acceptance.

For inspiration and writing topics, you may also visit: www.metajournals.com, a "clearinghouse" for journal writers, which provides a monthly newsletter and writing ideas.

Getting Started

4

Selecting the tools and materials for journal writing is a very personal process. Fortunately, there are no right or wrong choices. The best way to begin is to see how you respond to options such as a loose-leaf binder, a blank book covered in velvet or leather, a lined pad, or sheets of artist's paper. Which of these speaks to you? And how do you feel about a pen versus a computer?

Unless you find that a word processing program significantly aids the flow of your writing, try to resist composing your entries on a computer because handwriting offers many significant advantages. The words you write, your "marks," are as unique as your fingerprints. The shape of your letters, the slant of your words, the way your sentences stretch across the page provide additional clues to your state of mind. For instance, when you're stressed, rushed, or excited, does your writing become uneven and less legible? During times of calm control, is each of your letters more precisely formed? When you feel burdened and unhappy, do your words slant downward? These visual clues to your identity deepen the content of your writing. They make each journal entry more personal and expressive.

The writing instrument you choose will make a difference too. Choose a pen that fits comfortably in your hand and has a good weight. This might be your favorite

Handwriting Analysis

Emotional factors affect the formation, spacing, and stroke of written words. For this reason, experts believe that exaggerations in the formation of words suggest similar exaggerations in the writer's personality. The study of this connection is called graphology.

Graphologists analyze several areas of writing, including: the upper middle, and lower zones of a letter; line slope; writing slant; the pressure of the pen; ability to stay on the line; line thickness; spacing between letters, words, and lines; letter shapes; lead-in and ending strokes; speed of writing; rhythm of the group of letters or words; and the connectedness of the letters. Another key element is size. Size projects the writer's feelings of self-importance and self-esteem. Individually, these handwriting characteristics provide clues to the writer's personality, but they need to be combined with each other for an accurate evaluation. For more information, contact the National Society for Graphology at the address and phone number in the resource list at the end of this chapter.

brand of pen from high school, a novelty pen from a friend, or perhaps a beautiful fountain pen you found at a flea market. Some pens make writing easier because they glide across the paper. Try out your pen and paper combination to see what's best for you.

"Graphology, when practiced by a well-trained professional, offers the most direct and in-depth method of determining a writer's character, . . . understanding his or her behavior, and of observing the various developmental stages in which the writer may have encountered difficulties in early childhood, thereby possibly affecting his or her emotional status in later years.

Psychologists and other therapists find graphology to be an invaluable aid . . . since deep-seated problems . . . can readily be observed in the client's handwriting. Since graphology deals with every aspect of human life, it is used by . . . any person who is simply seeking better self-understanding."

—JANICE KLEIN, MANHATTAN HANDWRITING CONSULTANT

Just be sure to use a pen, not a pencil. After all, ink has a permanent quality and the point of writing a journal is to preserve who you are right now. This is why you must leave what you write intact and resist the urge to erase or edit. Also, consider the color ink you use. There are many choices. You can start with basic blue or black, or try more vivid colors to express your mood. The idea is to use whatever will enhance the power of your words.

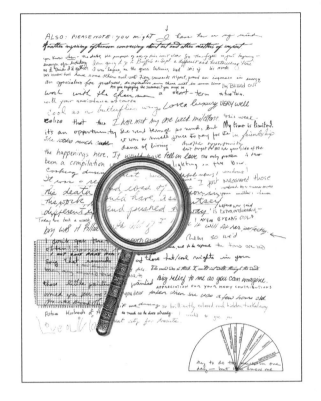

A study on graphology
Graphology, © Lois Guarino, 1997, courtesy of Robert Mann Gallery, NYC

Your Writing Environment

Once you've selected your tools, you need to find a writing retreat that suits you best. Fortunately, there is no "correct" location for writing. Some people prefer to be indoors working at a desk, sitting in a chair, or propped up in bed. Others are inspired by public places like a local park or favorite coffeehouse. Wherever you end up, two concerns should dictate your location: privacy and comfort.

Privacy means different things to different people. For some writers, it signifies a calm, quiet place where they can be alone. By contrast, fellow journalists might prefer an unoccupied corner of a large museum or anywhere they can be inspired by the buzz of daily life as long as it's not too distracting and there are no prying eyes. Wherever you stake your claim, you may find that using the same location consistently helps you establish a rhythm in your journal-writing routine. Just be sure to have your writing materials on hand and to surround yourself with things that put you at ease and help you focus.

For instance, if you're easily distracted, hang up a DO NOT DISTURB sign or simply don't answer the door during your private journal-writing time. You can also turn off your phone or let the answering machine catch your calls. These steps will help you concentrate, and concentration will enhance your experience on every level.

Beginnings

Many people start each journal-writing session with a ritual. They read an affirmation, pray, visualize, or light a candle to help them focus and eliminate mental distractions. Other people dive right into the backwaters of their life. If you're ready to take the plunge, one way to begin is with a regular routine like writing two or three pages a day even if you don't have anything to say.

In fact, if you don't have anything to say, make this the topic of your writing and don't worry about it. Eventually more ideas will come. They'll come because just finishing the task and making journal writing part of your daily routine sets up a new habit. Once the habit is ingrained, you will write in your journal. Scientific studies

Eliminating Mental Distractions

If you're so distracted you can't write, then write about your distractions. Start by putting a mundane pad of paper next to your journal. As you try to write entries and your mind insists on dictating the grocery list, enumerating errands, and other flotsam and jetsam, write it all down on the pad, then go back to your journal. No matter how many times you get distracted, keep going back. Eventually your mind will give up so you can move ahead and you'll have both your journal entries and the week's grocery list to show for it!

Beginning Your Journal in Childhood

Use five sentences to describe yourself at five years old, five sentences to describe yourself at ten years old, then at fifteen, twenty, and so on up to your present age. What did others—teachers, relatives, neighbors—say about you at these ages? How did your personal myth begin, develop, and grow? Is your family's interpretation of this myth still accurate? Is yours? Have other family members followed in your footsteps?

Communications teacher Shelly Carlson uses this exercise with her students and herself. She says, "I was very accident-prone and had lots of injuries. I have a nephew who's the same way. When he started having accidents, my family started calling him by my name. This, of course, has given us a bond and I first recognized this in my journal."

This exercise can help you decode myths about your family and yourself. It can assist you in deciphering social dynamics, working your way through holiday angst, and discovering truths and falsehoods. Whichever of these items you choose to tackle, childhood will give you plenty to write about.

show it takes thirty days of conscious, repetitive behavior for a new habit to become part of everyday life.

If two or three pages a day seems daunting, there are other ways to begin. Judith Taylor, a teacher at Northwestern University, writes that you don't always have to compose long passages because a journal welcomes idea fragments, single words, and incomplete thoughts, all of which can be insightful. Taylor suggests stories, images, artifacts, and visual aids to inspire creativity and release emotions. You can even use a piece of food and write about the taste, memories, or experiences associated with it.

Other options are to list daily events in chronological order and examine their meaning; describe an object or your physical surroundings through each of your five senses; play music and write about it; reveal three secrets about yourself, three things you like about yourself, and three memories of childhood.

Other Ways to Start the Journal-Writing Process

✦ Open a book, let a page fall open, and write your response to whatever you read.

✦ Eat three foods. Describe everything about these foods including their taste, smell, texture, look, and how they sound when you bite in. This helps you write about being in the moment. Then move on to any memories or associations these foods have for you.

✦ Teacher Mary Lewis of the River Oaks Arts Writing Center in Oak Park, Illinois, suggests this scenario. Adopt a baby called Creativity and write about how you convince the social worker that you are the right parent. Discuss how you have to change your schedule to take care of this "baby" and how much the "baby" means to you.

✦ Define freedom, including characteristics of freedom, what it would take for you to be free, how you can make this come about, and how long it will take. Now meditate on freedom. See yourself flying in a free, open space. How does it feel? Is your perceived lack of freedom due to a lack of time? Can you create moments of freedom for your mind, such as when you're doing some mindless, mundane task or when you're in transit? Write it down.

✦ Write about current events, politics, or what's going on in your community. You never know, says Loretta Pyrdek, when you are going to be a witness to history and your entries will be of value to future generations.

Loretta Pyrdek, adjunct faculty member at Chicago City Colleges, tells her students to write about the three Ps: problems, puzzles, and passions—that is, things they want to resolve, things that make them curious, and things they're crazy about. The three Ps might be a good place for you to start too, and you can write about these topics in as broad or narrow a way as you wish.

Another recommendation from Pyrdek is to set up a mirror, study your reflection, and describe what you see. Focus on the connections between your outer and inner self. Be forewarned, at first this might be uncomfortable. "There is so much resistance to exploring our interiority," Pyrdek says, "but eventually writing a self-portrait can create a breakthrough that is flowing and reflective. You will lose your self-consciousness, access your deeper thoughts, and foster a more reflective view of life. This is not only emotionally therapeutic, it improves your skills and self-confidence as a writer."

From a Single Word

Once you're feeling confident, you may find that a torrent of words pours out onto the first page of your journal, but if the idea of a torrent is too overwhelming, there are other ways to start.

Omega instructor Linda Trichter Metcalf, Ph.D., and her partner Tobin Simon, Ph.D., co-directors of the Proprioceptive Writing Center in New York, call their form of personal writing Proprioceptive Writing®. Metcalf describes Proprioceptive Writing as an expressive therapy that uses writing to explore the psyche by taking the emphasis off writing and focusing it on the experience of inner hearing, "the key to feeling and the doorway to self-knowledge." Proprioceptive Writing can be practiced alone or in groups.

In Proprioceptive Writing, the writer creates a safe space where she is free from outside interruption for periods of twenty-five minutes. In these sessions, Metcalf says, "Your phone is literally and figuratively off the hook." Mythically, you write in sacred time and space by ritualizing the setting: white unlined paper, Baroque music, candles. Within this cocoon, the writer learns to slow thought-flow down to the rhythms of speech and to track it in writing to its source in emotion and story.

The Mozart Effect

Studies prove that classical music stimulates intellectual and creative development. According to Don Campbell, author of *The Mozart Effect,* this can be particularly effective with children and infants.

Beginning Your Journal with Alphapoems

Kathleen Adams, M.A., LPC, of the Center for Journal Therapy in Colorado, uses Alphapoems to inspire her students in the journal-writing process. The first step is to pick a subject, such as a feeling, mood, an issue, task, a person, an event, or a check-in. Adams describes a check-in as what's going on with you right now, where you are, or what you want. The second step is to write a poem about your subject in which each successive line begins with the next letter of the alphabet. Adams says to work quickly to maximize creativity and unexpected results. She also says it's perfectly acceptable to use "xceptions for xtra-hard letters." Here's an example from an alphapoem by Adams entitled "Things I Love."

Angel cards,
Blistering hot August days
Cooled by a/Dip in the pool.
Energetic
Friends
Giggling
Heartily.
I love hot fudge sundaes, and
Juicy watermelon eaten over the
Kitchen sink.
Love letters.
Moments captured in photos or prose, the
Noisy-ness of nieces,
Orange blossom bubble bath and
Petrified wood forests.
Quarantined weekends alone, just for me.
Resting, reading, relaxing.

Summer's long days.
Turned into autumn's crispy nights.
Unwrapped gifts.
Victories triumphant.
Wild-mind writing,
eXceptional events,
Yearly trips to Taos—
Zowie! I'm in love.

To accomplish this feat, Proprioceptive Writing uses a tool known as the "proprioceptive question," or the PQ, which asks "What do I mean by?" With the aid of this mantralike question, the writer unpacks the personal experience encoded in her language. The readiness to ask the PQ focuses attention, heightens listening powers, and develops what Metcalf calls the auditory imagination. When the Write ends, four final questions provide further openings: "Thoughts heard but not written?" "How do I feel now?" "What story am I telling?" "Directions for future Writes?" Respond to these questions in writing. Read the results aloud. Then place it in your Proprioceptive Writing folder.

The text that Proprioceptive Writing produces is called a "Write," which like a dream can be analyzed by oneself or used to focus a therapy session. Proprioceptive Writing is a liberating, expressive method for both nonwriters who wish to write, as well as for writers facing psychological difficulties that impede their work. It provides a rich source of raw material for anyone interested in writing for publication and is an infallible method of problem-solving.

Metcalf and Simon—who have been teaching their form of process-writing since 1976—assert that Proprioceptive Writing unburdens the mind, resolves emotional conflict, enlivens the imagination, and integrates thinking and feeling. Regular practice results in sharper clarity; sustained focus; increased awareness and self-confidence; greater spontaneity, and a sense of growing intelligence and burgeoning creativity. As they remind their students, these benefits are the rewards of a happy addiction to daily practice.

The Time of Your Life

In our frantic society you need to catch moments whenever you can. This might mean keeping your journal with you and writing whenever opportunity permits, such as during your lunch break, while waiting in the doctor's office, or during the fifteen sacred minutes between the time your seven-year-old goes to school and the time your four-year-old wakes up.

One seventeenth-century author and mother of twelve handled it this way. She kept a bowl of water and a washcloth next to her whenever she was writing. If her children approached, they knew they would have their face and hands scrubbed before they could interrupt. Is it any surprise that the number of interruptions declined or that she had the cleanest kids in town?

Whether you choose to set aside cleanly chiseled out time or to write in odd moments, just practicing the discipline of writing is what's important. It's also important to give your journal your complete attention, what the Buddhists call "mindfulness," in order to derive the full benefit for the energy expended. After all, what you get out of your journal will be directly proportionate to what you put in.

If you put enough of yourself in, you'll increase your tolerance for healthy risks. Just starting a journal and getting to know yourself is an act of confidence that can carry over to other areas of your life. Your journal can also teach you additional life lessons, like how to play. Northwestern University instructor Judith Taylor describes this as the fine line between taking your entries seriously but not taking yourself seriously. Taylor also notes that you'll learn how to improvise on any topic and "to think of how you can do it differently next time." This builds flexibility, which might be valuable in your relationships. Last but not least, beginning a journal boosts your ego. Far from being self-indulgent, personal writing is a way to care for yourself and tend to your emotional and physical needs. Doing so benefits not only you but everyone you care about and is an excellent reason to begin.

If You Can't Write Every Day

Editor and teacher Mary Lewis says it's perfectly reasonable not to write every day. If you get busy with other things, are bored, or aren't getting enough from your journal, it doesn't mean you're not a good journalist. "Absence in a journal is normal," says Lewis in a recent interview. "It doesn't go anywhere and will be there when you need it."

Instructor Judith Taylor agrees. "Writing in a journal isn't about scheduling fifteen minutes a day or always doing it first thing in the morning . . . there's no need to feel guilty."

TO LEARN MORE ABOUT STARTING A JOURNAL, READ:

Baldwin, Christina. *One to One: Self-Understanding Through Journal Writing* (New York: Evans & Company, 1991).

Cameron, Julia. *The Artist's Way* (New York: Tarcher/Perigee, 1992).

Goldberg, Natalie. *Writing Down the Bones—Freeing the Writer Within* (Boston: Shambhala, 1986).

For more information contact:

The National Association for Graphology
250 West 57th Street, Room 1228A
New York, New York 10107
212-265-1148

For more information on the Center for Journal Therapy, contact:

Kathleen Adams, M.A., LPC, Director
The Center for Journal Therapy
12477 West Cedar Drive, Suite 102
Lakewood, Colorado 80228
888-421-2298

5.
Approaches to Writing

It's a rare person who comes to journal writing knowing exactly what she wants to say and how she wants to say it. For most people, including many veteran writers, the blank page or screen is intimidating. This is true whether it's the first time you sit down to write or every time you pick up a pen. Whatever the case, learning different approaches can expand your ability to communicate and help you build a storehouse of methods to overcome writer's block and other concerns.

In this chapter you'll be introduced to a broad sampling of exercises that will allow you to try your hand at different ways of writing. You'll also learn about writing techniques and tips from some of the country's foremost teachers and experts. You can sample all their methods, zero in on one which is a great fit, or customize different approaches to create a totally new way of working that suits your individual needs. This chapter will help you navigate the choices, but don't be discouraged if the process includes some trial and error. This exploration is part of your inward journey, and you will get to know yourself better as you undertake the process.

Surprisingly, journal writing as a documented means to inner discovery has only a brief history. Even though people have been writing journals for centuries, books, lectures, and seminars on the topic, as well as journal keeping as an assignment from a therapist have surfaced only in the last sixty years. The earliest documented cases are Jungian therapists assigning journal and dream diaries to their patients in the late 1920s and early 1930s. Other journal-writing techniques grew out of graduate school seminars and university research conducted in the last half of the twentieth century. The work of psychologist Ira Progoff, Ph.D., and educator Christina Baldwin, which will be discussed later in this chapter, stems from these workshop and university settings.

In addition, two influential approaches appeared in the 1970s from Morton Kelsey and Barbara Sher. Kelsey was a writer and teacher who compiled a journal of daily devotions, prayers, music, and his responses to the power of these spiritual elements. By contrast, therapist and career counselor Barbara Sher advocated a highly practical approach. She suggested using your journal to define who you are, to write a wish list clarifying your goals, to craft entries that plot a path toward those goals, and to create an action plan. Both methods were widely publicized and struck a chord with the reading public. As a result, Kelsey and Sher inspired many contemporary teachers and writers working in different areas, including the creative journal.

Writing the Creative Journal

The creative journal is a place to capture, nurture, and express ideas. These can be inspirations for a story, a piece of music, a recipe, a fresh approach to teaching, nurturing a relationship, or anything you like. In fact, anything and everything you do benefits from creativity. Keeping this spirit energized is key to a healthy, balanced lifestyle. This is why you can use the creative journal to explore many topics and in so doing create a place where unformed concepts can begin to take shape.

Bringing new concepts and ideas into a physical dimension is one important reason people take the creative approach. It doesn't matter if these ideas never go beyond the written page. Why? Just by writing your creative ideas down, you connect with your higher self, experience wholeness and life-affirming potential. Best of all, you don't have to be an artist to do this.

In *Wild Mind, Living the Writer's Life*, teacher Natalie Goldberg shows you how to make the most of this personal creative power. She starts with simple exercises to help you overcome procrastination and writer's block, then explains how to squeeze in time for writing among your daily responsibilities. To help you achieve this, Goldberg advocates certain rules for writing practice. These are probably unlike any "rules" you've followed before because they are designed to help you break free from the constraints of your conscious mind. First, says Goldberg, "keep your hand moving, be specific, lose control, don't think, don't worry about punctuation, spelling, and grammar, feel free to write the worst junk, go for the jugular." Goldberg says that if you apply these guidelines, you will write more loosely, making it easier to address difficult subjects.

Creative journal expert Julia Cameron, author of *The Artist's Way, A Spiritual Path to Higher Creativity,* agrees. She says "by moving my hand across the page I move the hand of the universe across my life. Such movement can help bring your life into align-

An Interview with a Student of Julia Cameron's

In the following interview, Carol Kravetz, a production coordinator for TV and film based in Hollywood, California, describes her experience using *The Artist's Way.*

Q: What is your personal history with journal writing and how did you come to *The Artist's Way?*
A: I have been keeping a journal on and off for many, many years but it was sporadic and seemingly without purpose except to vent my personal horrors. . . . I found I wanted to expand my creative horizons and had heard so many good things about Julia Cameron's *The Artist's Way* that I decided to try it.

Q: Describe your experiences with this method.
A: Ms. Cameron gives you daily and weekly tasks for a twelve-week period in order to hone your writing, thinking, and artistic skills. The main task is writing three pages a day, every day. I do not consider myself a writer by any means.

Q: Since you don't consider yourself a writer, how did this work out?
A: I had a difficult time writing three pages a day. Some days I'd stare at that gall-darn blank page and have nothing in my brain to write. There were times all I would write . . . was blah, blah, blah, or "I have nothing to write" a dozen times until my hand got sore. I seemed to do well up to a page and a half . . . then the words just fail me. . . . But I seem to be stuck on the idea of pen to paper being the only way to really get your most personal inner thoughts communicated. . . .

Guide for Living the Creative Process Day by Day

Dan Wakefield, a well-known teacher and author of *Creating from the Spirit,* offers these steps for bringing more creativity into your daily life.

- Wake up to music and birdsong, not buzzers.
- Inscribe the day. Determine what you want to do with it rather than what it will do to you.
- Sit down to breakfast at a beautiful table, pray, and eat slowly.
- Visualize your work.
- Play a new role.
- Take a walk, practice yoga.
- Take exercise breaks from writing.

ment." What Cameron means is that writing lets you see how experiences shape your life and how you fit into the bigger world picture. It's a way of seeing your purpose, understanding your challenges, and directing your energy.

Cameron has two essential exercises to help you achieve this aligned state. The first is Morning Pages, which aids you in clearing away distractions, mental clutter, and preoccupations at the start of the day. Here's how it works.

When you roll out of bed, put your pen to paper and write three stream-of-consciousness pages every day. If nothing comes to mind, write anyway; you can even write "I have nothing to say." If it's helpful, keep a file of drawings, letters, or articles about things that interest you. When you're stuck for what to say in the Morning Pages, pull something out of your file and write a response as a way to keep your creative juices flowing and establish a writing habit.

"It is the imagination that helps us find meaning and beauty in our lives. . . . we are alive or dead according to the condition of our souls."

—CAROL S. PEARSON

> "Courage is necessary to creativity, but too often we confuse courage with comfort."
>
> —JULIA CAMERON

The second exercise Cameron uses is the Artist's Date. This is a date you make with yourself for a specific time, place, and activity. Whether it's something you've done before or something totally new, the point of the activity is to recharge your creative batteries. You can go to a movie or art exhibit, listen to music, play with your child, or engage in the delights of aimless wandering. Whatever your choice, the activity should be something that refreshes your spirit and inspires your imagination.

With that imagination, you can create new solutions, craft innovations, and reinvent yourself. Whether you adopt the techniques of Natalie Goldberg, Julia Cameron, or someone else, or come up with an approach of your own, the creative journal empowers you and boosts your self-confidence. You feel more fully alive and able to act on your potential not only for journal writing but for life.

Using Your Journal to Create Characters and Tell Stories

There's the romantic you and the practical you; the conservative you and the radical you; old you and young you; you the parent and you the child; and all the yous in between. These "yous" represent different parts of your personality. Although sometimes these parts are in conflict, that's not as bad as it seems. The fact that we're all pulled by different aspects of our personalities can make for some fascinating journal entries, especially if you think of these parts as characters. In fact, when you write about an internal tug-of-war, your journal may read like a novel complete with fully developed plots and settings, heroes and villains. This can be quite intriguing.

Therapist Deena Metzger has developed an approach that lets you capture these characters, which she calls splits, and understand them more fully. To begin the process, list your inner conflicts. Select one that is particularly pressing. For example,

Using Fiction Techniques to Be the Hero
of Your Own Life Story

Christopher Vogler, a teacher and former script consultant with Disney, writes that certain basic characters and structural patterns from myths form the basis of modern storytelling. With the following exercise, you can use some of the elements Vogler identifies to write your true life story as a heroic journey. Be sure to include real people and real incidents, then follow these steps in your journal:

1. Describe your ordinary, everyday world.

2. Describe the call to adventure that changes your world.

3. What did you learn on your journey? Describe this in your journal.

maybe you're a grown woman but around your mother you act like a child. Now, choose a personal incident that illustrates this split, an incident in which you responded to your mother with one part of yourself, the child, while suppressing another part of yourself, the adult. Perhaps this conflict arose when you bought your new car or took a new job. Whatever it was, write the story twice, counsels Metzger, once from your inner child's point of view and once from your perspective as an adult.

As you examine your entries, you may discover that this split represents an internal wound that never healed. To move toward healing, examine how the characters live within you now. Use your journal to document when the split is most likely to occur, to describe events that precede the split, to explore all sides of the issue, and to give each character a distinctive voice. One way to do the latter, writes Metzger, is to imagine an accident and describe each character's response to the trauma. This approach can help you differentiate between the characters in your head and ensure that each has a unique identity.

You may want to consider Metzger's technique or those like it if you are using your journal as the basis for fiction or want to turn your entries into plays, poems, songs, or other creative work. A story/character approach creates cohesion for your characters and for you as you listen to every part of yourself.

An Archetypal Approach to Writing a Journal

An archetype is the original model that sets the standard for others of its kind. It also represents certain universal truths so it's easy to recognize. In other words, you'll know an archetype when you see one. After all, don't you always recognize the villain by his slick smile and two-timing ways? The nice guy by his modesty and sincerity? The warrior queen by her sense of justice and inner strength? You can use these and other archetypes as a way to approach writing in your journal.

They're helpful because they give you a starting point to define your own behavior. With an archetype as a guide, you can use traditions passed down in myths and literature to formulate a personal code of conduct and devise a direction for any given situation. Researcher Carol S. Pearson has created just such a system based on a twenty-year study she began in graduate school. Her archetypes include the innocent, the orphan, the warrior, the caregiver, the seeker, the destroyer, the lover, the creator, the ruler, the magician, and the fool.

At different moments in life we all find ourselves playing these various roles. By using archetypes as a guide, we can handle these roles a little better and learn more about who we are and who we want to be. For instance, if you've lost your job, you might feel orphaned. As an orphan you want to regain your sense of safety and security, but you fear that you will be exploited before you ever reach this goal. Your response to this fear is a feeling of powerlessness and a deep desire for rescue, but your task, says Pearson, is to process the fear and pain and seek help from others. In so doing you, the orphan, learn empathy, interdependence, and get a valuable reality check.

Similarly, if you've asked for a divorce, you might feel like a destroyer. As a destroyer, you seek metamorphosis and positive change in your life, but you fear that change means the end of something rather than a new beginning. For instance, after a divorce, you may be afraid no one will ever love you again. As a destroyer, your response to this fear is to destroy or be destroyed, and you may lash out angrily at those around you as a way of defending yourself and hiding your fears. Your task in this archetypal role is to accept

Writing as a Wild Woman—A Female Archetypal Approach

"We are filled with a longing for the wild," writes Jungian analyst Clarissa Pinkola Estés, "but there are few culturally sanctioned antidotes for this yearning. We were taught to feel shame for such a desire. The shadow of the Wild Woman still lurks behind us during our days and in our nights. The Wild Woman archetype sheathes the alpha matrilineal being."

Where the Wild Woman once represented a dynamic, powerful female force, it has now been reduced to the stereotype of the evil stepmother or bitch-goddess so popular in movies. This perversion of the archetype, writes Pinkola Estés, impacts women's well-being because it denies an essential part of the female self. Fortunately, you can recapture your Wild Woman by working with this archetype in your journal. Begin with the following steps:

1. Examine the role of the Wild Woman in fairy tales and myths.

2. Write a straightforward account of an incident where you suppressed your Wild Woman side.

3. Now write about the same incident as a fairy tale in which your Wild Woman is set free to behave as she wishes. Examine the outcome.

4. Consider how you might apply aspects of your Wild Woman side to be more assertive and true to yourself. Examine this in your journal entries.

your mortality and the fact that you couldn't make your marriage work. Your reward for going through this process is greater acceptance and humility.

Ultimately, using archetypes as a guide for your journal entries can provide direction and aid you in your personal transformation, especially if you accompany this approach with meditation, prayer, and positive visualization.

Writing About Milestones in Your Life

Many people associate the word "milestone" with a birth, death, wedding, divorce, relocation, or retirement. Although these are all marker events, a milestone is something more. A milestone is an event that changes your life. It spins you around 360 degrees and alters your way of thinking, your relationships, your physical or spiritual being. For instance, maybe your ninth birthday passed uneventfully but later that same year, your teacher praised you for being the best student in class. Suddenly you became more confidant and outgoing, developing personality traits that have helped you blossom into the person you are today. The experience was a milestone because it changed your life in a significant way.

Whatever your milestones are, writing about them helps you determine what is important in your life. It helps you understand what formed the person you are and explains the path you've chosen. Susan Wittig Albert, teacher, novelist, and originator of the Story Circle Journal, suggests several life milestones to consider for your entries. Some include:

- ✦ Soul Mates: who your soul mates are and why; the meaning of love and how you express it in your life.

- ✦ Writing Home: whether there's anyplace like home; what home means in emotional terms; how you have provided a home for yourself and others; if you are at home with yourself; whether you consider the world your home; how your notion of home has changed over the years.

- ✦ Valley of Shadows: your dark side; what you've learned from this part of yourself; how it has made you stronger and wiser; what sustains you when you pass through dark times; how you move from darkness into light.

- ✦ Common Interests, Common Causes: where you fit in the world; how you interact with your family and others; your place in the universe.

You can use Wittig Albert's approach or organize your milestone entries in a different way. For instance, you can arrange them chronologically or create a list of impact

> "I have discovered in the course of my journey that life and psychic growth move
> in cycling spiral rings of descent and ascent. Every new growth in myself has been
> preceded by a descent of the seed into the dark ground."
>
> —LINDA SHIERSE LEONARD, WRITER, TEACHER

statements in which you describe how various people have affected your life. Another option is writing about milestones in the lives of those connected to you. In addition, you can use your entries to mark stages of illness and wellness, professional passions and triumphs, or memories and reminiscences. Whatever you choose, the milestone approach is an opportunity to pave your way back to the past and forward to the future.

A Letter-Writing Approach

When you get a letter, writes teacher, trainer, and motivational consultant Joyce Chapman, you are instantly transported to the writer's world, to his or her experience and physical reality. You can capture this same feeling by writing letters to yourself or other people.

Filling your journal with such personal correspondence organizes events for your mind's eye and makes it easier to see the cause-and-effect sequence of your actions. In addition, because a letter approach is very intimate, it loosens up your style so it's more comfortable for you to write. Best of all, you don't have to send this correspondence unless you want to.

To use the letter-writing approach, start by compiling a list of people you want to write to. You might want to communicate with family members, elderly relatives, a friend who is special to you, someone you've lost touch with, people you would like to thank, or even yourself.

Once you have your list, there are several kinds of letters you can compose. For instance, you can use a milestone letter to commemorate an important event. Such letters help you preserve your perception of a special point in time. You can also use them as a gauge to check your position in the future.

Another option is the release letter. Release letters allow you to vent and express your deepest emotions, especially the emotions you're not ready to share. Chapman states these "free up buried energy, allowing you to think and feel things through." Just remember that release letters don't always lead to resolution. They do, however, lead to change because they help you clean out negative emotions and stop these feelings from impacting your life. It's your decision whether to actually send a release letter or not.

Similarly, you can choose whether to send a wisdom letter or not. You may want to write a wisdom letter if you find yourself dealing with a situation that causes you great difficulty or personal strife. Wisdom letters move you beyond anger and revenge to unexpected clarity and, writes Chapman, "allow you to speak from a deeper, more objective place using words to bring healing and release."

You might write a wisdom letter if your family is divided by addiction, illness, divorce, or other issues. It's a good place to start a dialogue on these subjects because wisdom letters allow you to express your deep love, concern, worries, or thoughts about behavior you don't understand.

In addition to wisdom letters, you can also use your journal to express thanks. Thank-you letters show your deep appreciation to those people—living or dead—who have made a difference in your life. You can even write thank-you letters to yourself in

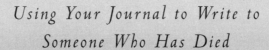

Using Your Journal to Write to Someone Who Has Died

In *Understanding, Coping, and Growing Through Grief,* Theresa S. Schoeneck of The Hope for the Bereaved, Inc., in Syracuse, New York, suggests these starting places if you want to write a letter to someone who has died.

+ A special memory that I have about you

+ What I miss most about you and our relationship

+ What I wish I'd said or hadn't said

+ What I'd like to ask you

+ What I wish we'd done or hadn't done

+ What I've had the hardest time dealing with

+ Ways in which you will continue to live on in me

+ Special ways I have for keeping my memories of you alive

acknowledgment of your own achievements and the difference you've made to others. This giving of thanks is one of life's profound experiences. Whether you do it in your journal, verbally, or through prayer and meditation, gratitude fills you with positive life energy and strengthens your connection to the universe. It frees you up to focus on new emotional, spiritual, and physical terrain so you can make it part of your conscious life.

Approaching Your Journal Through a Group

Some people are more productive when they work with a journal-writing group. A group can provide support, encouragement, and a sense of security as you move into unknown territory.

Writing Helps Heal Grief

Shelley Tatelbaum, certified grief therapist and founder/director of the Center for Grief, Loss, and Life Transition in Poughkeepsie, New York, had a client who was trying to cope with guilt over her sister's suicide. Tatelbaum advised the client to write a letter to her sister. In the letter, the client expressed the depth of feelings she had about the death. On the next page of her journal the client wrote back to herself in her sister's voice. This journal correspondence was repeated at least twice until all the feelings were exchanged. "This is a beneficial technique for people who find themselves in situations without closure, where unfinished business prevents healing. Carrying on a conversation between you and the person you are grieving over can have a tremendous therapeutic effect. It lowers repression and a flow of unconscious material emerges," Tatelbaum explains.

If you choose to work with a group, teacher Christina Baldwin says it is extremely important for you to respect each other's personal privacy and remember that what is shared in the writing circle must stay within that circle. Members should also learn to listen without giving advice and to pass tissues, not judgments, during emotional moments.

Once these ground rules are set, your group can experiment with different writing techniques. Whatever method you use, it's helpful to maintain silence while people are working. When the writing time is up, ask for volunteers to read and encourage group members to listen carefully without offering critiques. This creates a secure setting where you can build self-confidence, nurture each other, and expand your comfort level.

After three to six months, your group can do a self assessment to decide how things are going. This evaluation provides members with a graceful exit point, should they wish to move on, and it brings in new energy as other writers replace them. Don't let this natural evolution distress you. It simply means people are growing and your group is working as it should. The blend of writing and talking, of fresh ideas de-

"Honor the writing. Honor the silence. Honor your life stories and you will be fine."
—CHRISTINA BALDWIN

veloped through exercises and new members, can stimulate everyone and provide paths to self-knowledge you might not have reached on your own.

The Intensive Journal Approach

One of the most famous of all journal-writing methods is an approach called the Intensive Journal. The Intensive Journal is a structured method of journal writing that uses logs and a feedback section for personal and spiritual growth. Its inventor, Dr. Ira Progoff, a student of Jung's, writes in his book, *At a Journal Workshop: Writing to Access the Power of the Unconscious and Evoke Creative Ability*, "The Intensive Journal . . . is . . . designed to provide an instrument and techniques by which persons can discover within themselves the resources they did not know they possessed. It is to enable them to draw the power of deep contact out of the actual experiences of their lives . . . recognize their own identity and harmonize it with the larger identity of the universe as they experience it. Where they had negated themselves, they can, by means of their Intensive Journal work, give their lives full value."

To discover this value using Progoff's method, you keep a number of logs including the Period Log; the Daily Log; the History Log; the Meditation Log; the Dream Log; and the Twilight Imagery Log. Twilight imagery is a collection of images, impressions, emotions, and symbols about your life that come to you through your senses and through conscious inward perceptions. Next, you write a feedback section that is used in conjunction with these logs.

In the feedback section, you use your logs to "bring . . . transformations of awareness" and focus on "inner movements of experience." Ultimately, says Progoff, this process generates " . . . the energy that carries . . . life toward its meaningful unfolding."

The Intensive Journal method may help you live more meaningfully now. Working through this process may help you establish continuity, direction, and a sense of forward motion. It may also provide some perspective on your personal history, help you refocus, live in the moment, and experiment with your potential. According to Progoff, this happens because the Intensive Journal helps you develop whole life perspective and position yourself "between the past and the future in such a way that . . . current actions . . . support . . . new potentials in . . . life."

If you choose to experience the Intensive Journal approach in a workshop setting, the potential, process, and intent are essentially the same. You still work as an individual with safety and privacy guaranteed. The workshops are taught by certified instructors in a group setting. No one judges or comments on your work and it is safe to be honest. It may be a good way for you to overcome inertia, expand inner capacity, and develop spiritual awareness in a group setting.

A Physical Approach: Using Your Journal to Take Care of Your Body

Although many experts use journal writing for an exploration of the mind and spirit, you can also use your entries to explore your physical self. For instance, since the ideal body in Western culture is a young, slim body, the aging process poses a conflict for many people. If you're one of them, you might disassociate from your body, have trouble experiencing physical pleasure, or deny your corporal being as a source of wisdom and energy.

If this is happening to you, your journal can help you recover the joy and integrity of your physical being. Begin by asking yourself questions about your body. Write about your first physical memory, the body messages you got from your family, what your body was like as a child, whether your gender or appearance made you uncomfortable, how it felt to experience adolescence, and how others responded to your body.

Now write about your expectations of the aging process. Include what you look forward to and what you dread. Then stand naked in front of a mirror and, as objectively as you can, describe what you see. You can also study the face of your same-sex parent or grandparent. How does she look to you? Does she feel good about her body? Does anything about that surprise you? Record your reactions, being careful to separate your objective observations from your subjective thoughts. Finally, decide what aspects of physical aging you can do something about and develop an action plan. For everything beyond your control, use your journal to work on acceptance and a positive frame of mind.

As you study these entries, you will uncover any false myths you've harbored about your physical being. You'll also be able to release yourself from what society thinks and accept your body as a healthy, wholesome place to live. This clarity will help you get beyond the clamor of cultural messages and see that the aging process is not a wasteland, just another step in the evolution of your authentic self.

One way you can reach this state is by using your journal to incorporate sacred pampering into your life. Sacred pampering is any highly valued, deeply respected experience that nurtures your body and soul, giving you happiness and inner peace.

To achieve these pampering experiences, writes Debrena Jackson Gandy, trainer, consultant, and keynote speaker, write a list of the things that bring you joy, both things from childhood and things you like as an adult. Then list your current priorities and the myths that are prevalent in your life. Do these two lists conflict? For instance, do you

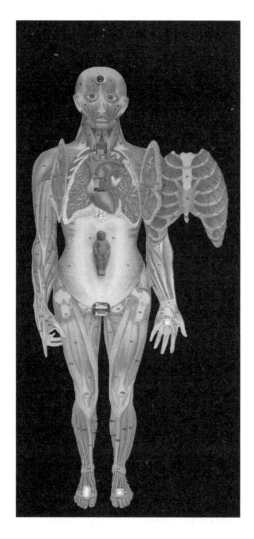

An anatomical photo-collage
Anatomy (fragment), © Lois Guarino, 1997,
courtesy of Robert Mann Gallery, NYC

"I think it is time . . . we stop denying our growing older and look at the actuality of our own experience and that of other women and men who have gone beyond denial to a new place in their sixties, seventies, and eighties."

—BETTY FRIEDAN, FEMINIST WRITER AND LEADER

want more time to yourself but say yes to every request and obligation? Once you see this problem, you can use your journal to begin to resolve it. Start by reframing any negative entries in positive words. For example, instead of writing "I have a weight problem," write "I have a weight challenge." This reframing will help you reconcile your conflicts, priorities, and myths with your sense of joy.

You can also transform your life if you use your entries to make peace with your physical self. Then you can celebrate this peace by building an altar, creating a sacred space where you can commune with your body, or learning to dance. Whatever you do, glory in your health and revel in the unique flesh that houses your life energy.

Writing the Spiritual Autobiography

Author China Galland says one of her first great spiritual awakenings took place when she visited the Grand Canyon. For Dan Wakefield, it happened when he faced personal tragedy. Like Wakefield and Galland, you may have life experiences in which you glimpse the face of a Higher Power and feel your spirit grow. The spiritual autobiography is the story of this very personal journey. It is a record of your spiritual history including events, revelations, prayers, devotions, meditations, questions, musings, and anything else that leads to the deepening of your soul.

Wakefield, a scriptwriter, teacher, and author, whose books include *Returning* and *The Story of Your Life: Writing a Spiritual Autobiography*, uses the spiritual autobiography to search for the values that form an ideal life. He has firsthand experience with this process. At age forty-eight, Wakefield left his home, a successful career, and his lover of seven years. He moved to Boston, ran out of money, faced the death of both parents, and confronted and healed his alcoholism, all in one year. Wakefield says he was saved by a class that taught him to use his journal as a spiritual autobiography.

You, too, may find the spiritual autobiography to be a powerful tool because it can help you learn forgiveness, gain inner peace, and leave behind whatever inhibits your spiritual growth. One way to approach it is like this. Start by defining what the

An Interview with Dan Wakefield

Teacher and author Dan Wakefield had this to say about the power of journal writing in his life.

Q: What was the moment of truth when you knew you had to change your life?
A: In *Returning*, I describe how, one balmy spring morning in Hollywood, a month or so before my forty-eighth birthday, I woke up screaming. I got out of bed, went into the next room . . . and screamed again. . . . It was a response to the reality that another morning had broken in a life I could only deal with sedated by wine, loud noise, moving images, and wired to electronic games that further distracted my fragmented attention from a growing sense of a blank, nameless pain in the pit of my very being, my most essential self.

Q: How did you choose journal writing, specifically the spiritual autobiography, to help you recover?
A: I took a course in church from my minister, Carl Scovel. It was an adult education class held in the living room of the King's Chapel parish house of a Unitarian church in Boston, where I had moved from Hollywood. The course was called Religious Autobiography and it asked you to trace the story of your life from a spiritual standpoint . . . it was a powerful process for me . . .

Q: What is the best way to approach the spiritual autobiography in a journal?
A: I believe the most valuable way to do autobiographical writing is in a community, not private musings as in journaling alone. Spiritual autobiography has more depth and you can share your life and insights with other people in a safe class setting. You may write alone as well as in class, but you share your story in a private group community setting.

word *spiritual* means to you. You can frame this definition in a specific religious structure or acknowledge a path beyond organized religion. Then draw a picture of the present to describe what's currently happening in your spiritual life. Write about what you've drawn, and if you choose, share it with others.

After sharing where you are in the present, go back to the past. Think about any childhood mentor, friend, or relative who served as a spiritual guide. Now move up through adolescence and young adult spiritual memories until you reach the present. This helps you trace your path and more clearly define the spirituality in your life. As part of this process, you might include entries about specific spiritual experiences and retreats, situations that put you in touch with a Higher Power, and how you translated these feelings into action. You might also look at pivotal events in your life from a universal perspective. What was the universe trying to teach you? Did you learn the lesson? Did you share it? Actualize it in your life? Are these spiritual lessons getting harder or easier? Whatever you write, be sure to give your entries a beginning, a middle, and an end. This gives your work shape, a sense of spiritual coherency, and completion.

Another way to use your journal for a sense of completeness is through spiritual mapping. Pioneered by teacher/author China Galland, *The Bond Between Women: A Journey to Fierce Compassion*, spiritual mapping encourages you to use your nonverbal skills to help visualize your soul's journey. Start by painting or drawing your entire spiritual life from beginning to end on a long piece of paper. This allows you to visually experience patterns and connections and trace your own spiritual timeline. Now describe these images in words in your journal.

Letting your thoughts flow from heart to hand to picture to word is an excellent way to record images and feelings you can't otherwise capture. By working back and forth, you will develop your own symbology and become more comfortable transcribing your spiritual journey onto the written page. You can even leave a few pages at the beginning of your journal blank, says Galland, so you can create an index of what's important and see spiritual patterns over time.

At some point, consider whether you wish to share these patterns with others on a similar quest. Sharing in a safe group setting can be an amazing spiritual catalyst that others can support and witness. Galland recommends undertaking this with a teacher, guide, or some form of community. "You need to have context as you probe, an anchor for your psyche," she says, "especially if you haven't much experience in dialoguing with your inner life. You need not embark alone."

And you are never alone when you keep a journal. Using these different approaches and tailoring them to your needs ensures that you will always have your most meaningful memories, your sharpest perceptions, and deepest spiritual self by your side. You will also have the foremost teachers and experts to guide you as you follow their methods and learn from their wisdom.

TO LEARN MORE ABOUT DIFFERENT APPROACHES TO JOURNAL WRITING, READ:

Baldwin, Christina. *One to One: Self-Understanding Through Journal Writing* (New York: Evans & Co., 1991).

Cameron, Julia. *The Artist's Way* (New York: Tarcher/Perigee, 1992).

Campbell, Joseph. *The Hero with a Thousand Faces* (Princeton, NJ: Princeton University Press, 1949; reissued 1990).

Chapman, Joyce. *Journaling for Joy* (North Hollywood, Calif.: Newcastle, 1991).

Clark, Kenneth. *Civilization* (New York: Harper & Row, 1969).

Dossey, Larry. *Recovering the Soul* (New York: Bantam Books, 1989).

Estés, Clarissa Pinkola. *Women Who Run with the Wolves* (New York: Ballantine Books, 1992).

Gandy, Debrena Jackson. *Sacred Pampering Principles: An African American Woman's Guide to Self-Care and Inner Renewal* (New York: William Morrow, 1997).

Goldberg, Natalie. *Wild Mind—Living the Writer's Life* (New York: Bantam Books, 1990).

Goldberg, Natalie. *Writing Down the Bones—Freeing the Writer Within* (Boston: Shambhala, 1986).

Goldstein, Joseph, and Jack Kornfield. *Seeking the Heart of Wisdom* (Boston: Shambhala, 1987).

Harding, M. Esther. *Woman's Mysteries Ancient and Modern* (New York: Harper Colophon, 1971).

Leonard, Linda Shierse. *On the Way to the Wedding* (Boston: Shambhala, 1986).

Leonard, Linda Schierse. *Witness to the Fire—Creativity and the Veil of Addiction* (Boston: Shambhala, 1989).

Metzger, Deena. *Writing from Your Life* (New York: Harper Collins, 1992).

Myss, Caroline. *Anatomy of the Spirit: The Seven Stages of Power and Healing* (New York: Random House, 1996).

Pearson, Carol S. *Awakening the Heroes Within: 12 Archetypes to Help Us Find Ourselves and Transform Our World* (San Francisco: Harper San Francisco, 1991).

Progoff, Ira. *At a Journal Workshop: Writing to Access the Power of the Unconscious and Evoke Creative Ability* (New York: Tarcher/Putnam, 1975).

Rainer, Tristine. *The New Diary: How to Use a Journal for Self-Guidance and Expanded Creativity* (New York: Tarcher, 1978).

Sher, Barbara, with Anne Gottlieb. *Wishcraft* (New York: Ballantine Books, 1983).

Spiegelman, J. Marvin, Pir Vilayat Khan, and Tasnim Fernandez. *Sufism, Islam, & Jungian Philosophy* (Scottsdale, Ariz.: Falcon Press, 1991).

Vogler, Christopher. *The Writer's Journey: Mythic Structure for Storytellers and Screenwriters* (Studio City, Calif.: Michael Wiese Productions, 1992).

Wakefield, Dan. *Creating from the Spirit* (New York: Damariscotta, 1996).

Wittig-Albert, Susan. *Writing from Life* (New York: Penguin Putnam, 1996).

FOR MORE INFORMATION ON THE PROGOFF
INTENSIVE JOURNAL METHOD, CONTACT:

Dialogue House
  1-800-221-5844
  80 East 11th Street, Suite 305
  New York, New York 10003-6008
  http://www.intensivejournal.org.

FOR JOURNAL WRITERS DEALING WITH
LOSS AS A SUBJECT, CONTACT:

Renew—Center for Personal Recovery, Journals for the Bereaved, at
  www.renew@mis.net

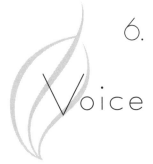

6.

Voice

Your voice is the way you choose to express yourself in your journal: your tone, attitude, choice of words, and point of view. We all use many different voices throughout the day, and this chorus can be helpful in the journal-writing process. Just as an actor takes on a role, you might take on a particular voice to understand a perspective or allow a different part of yourself to come through. You might use a positive, encouraging voice, as Natalie Goldberg recommends, to bolster your creative self; a judgmental voice, as Julia Cameron does, to assess an issue; or a voice of history, like Alex Haley, to speak to future generations.

In this chapter are some options for experimenting with different voices that best reflect your feelings, express your message, and communicate with a particular audience, even if the only person in that audience is you. We'll start with the autobiographic voice.

The Autobiographic Voice

If you are writing a diary, writes Tristine Ranier, teacher and director of the Center for Autobiographic Studies in Pasadena, California, you are writing in the "ever-mov-

> "We live the stories of our lives with such intensity and engagement that they are transparent to us. We eat, sleep, dream, breathe them. We are like fish swimming in the ocean. What fish imagines itself surrounded by water, or knows there are creatures that breathe a lighter, brighter air?"
>
> —SUSAN WITTIG ALBERT

ing present." By contrast, autobiographic writing is in retrospect. It is a voice of recollection in which you look back at your memories and use them to tell the story of your life.

Essentially, that story is a meaningful pattern of events in which you are the main character. Like any main character, you have clear-cut goals and desires. Your autobiography is the story of these desires, of what you wanted, how you struggled, and what you learned in the process. This makes the autobiography a tale of growth, a tale that proves that you are not engaged in aimless wandering but rather have a purpose to your life.

To write in the autobiographic voice, start by accessing your memories. There are many ways to do this. You can play music from an era you're trying to recall, make a favorite family recipe, or look at a photograph. You can also research the past by interviewing your relatives or using body memories, like that scar on your knee or the broken arm you got when you fell off your bike. Try writing about these memory fragments or capture your thoughts on a tape recorder and transfer them to your journal later. Just be sure to use all of your senses to make the memory come alive. Write in the present tense, adding movement and detail—physical, verbal, and emotional—then see what other recollections your memory fragment triggers and write about them in the same way.

As you do this, you will discover that your early perceptions and your mature observations overlap. Why? Because your memories aren't just about the past, they are about the past as seen from the present, with all the insight and perspective the intervening time offers. This is particularly true when you remember conflicts you have with yourself or others.

Conflicts are like an embroidery thread. They are the issues that keep resurfacing in your life, and they form the themes in your autobiographic journal. These themes

James Hillman's Acorn Theory

In his "acorn theory," psychoanalyst James Hillman says knowing your unique character can lead you to the intrinsic truth of your life. It can dispel the illusion that your personal history is "a series of accidents or calamities that wrongly formed you." In other words, the autobiographic voice can demonstrate that your life is your own creation. It is not the result of somebody else's whim but a reflection of your own choices, spiritual path, and conscious awareness.

might include relationships that need tending, issues you need to confront, or changes in your spirituality. Whatever the case, you may need to tie off these thematic threads so they don't disrupt the fabric of your life. Ranier states this is why you must read your life like a book and "ask what hidden significance . . . these characters and events have" for you.

Writing about your real experiences with real people can help you recall scenes you've forgotten, acknowledge special connections, and provide a structural framework. In addition, using actual dialogue and humor from your everyday life can make your autobiography compelling to read. It's even more readable if you reach for a sense of mystery and complexity that can deepen your entries. Essentially, this means approaching your story as literature.

A literary approach uses a classic structure to help you organize your thoughts and tell your story in a more powerful way. First, decide what you want to write about. Perhaps it's a pivotal event, a destination you reached, or a satisfying outcome you achieved. Next, identify the conflict in the situation. What happened the first time the conflict arose? Did it bring a particular problem to your attention? Did you know about this problem before? Now that you know, what do you want out of the situation? Who or what keeps you from getting it? Do you overcome these obstacles or not? How does it make you feel?

Next, move on to the event that turns your story in another direction. Ranier believes this takes place about two-thirds of the way to your conclusion and it comes right before the crisis. The crisis is your emotional low point or the point of greatest physical danger. It is the moment when the conflict with your adversary is at its most intense. The crisis leads to the climax, the point of decision or change when something—an old truth or dream—must die so something else, such as your future, can live. It is the moment when transformation takes place.

After transformation comes your conclusion: what you achieved, the knowledge you gained, how it changed you, and how you feel about the outcome. Last, explain why you wanted to capture this story in an autobiographic voice and if the literary structure helped you succeed.

While it's true that literary structure can empower your writing, it's also true that literary structure can be intimidating. You may feel blocked by a lack of language or form, but this can be overcome by prewriting in your journal. Prewriting means taking the time to define your desires before you write a chronology of events. This allows you to tap into your personal myths and decide what you want to write about. The process fertilizes both your mind and your journal for all kinds of autobiographic work, including the confession.

The Confession

The confession has a long and fascinating history. Ancient Egyptians confessed their good deeds in writing, then placed these texts on the chests of the dead as a passport to the next world. By contrast, many Christians thought it important to write their confessions before death so there would be time to repent. Augustine undertook this process by cataloging his sins in an autobiographic journal called *Confessions*. In his entries, the saint laments that his soul is in ruins and he asks God to help him rebuild his life. Augustine then used his journal to seek salvation, attain conversion, and self-healing. Other Christians used their journals in similar ways. Some of these famous, early confessional autobiographies include *The Revelation of St. John the Divine* and *The Lives of the Saints*.

Sainthood was apparently not what Jean-Jacques Rousseau had in mind when, in his secular autobiography, he confessed to thievery, bearing false witness, and consigning five of his children to a foundling home. Rousseau broke new ground in autobiographical frankness, and his influence can be seen to this day in sensational publications like *True Confessions* and *Real Romance* magazines, which have been popular since the 1940s.

Given these varied examples, how can you apply the confessional voice in your writing? One option is to use your journal for secular or spiritual housecleaning. Such cleaning may allow you to choose a new direction, forgive yourself and others, and reach a new level of spiritual grace.

Another way is to use the confessional voice to explore your family relationships. Researcher Maggie Scarf, a past fellow at the Center for Advanced Study in Behavioral Sciences at Stanford University, writes that families are intensely emotional social systems, even if they appear to display no emotion at all. Within this system, you learn a particular set of rules about your own and other people's behavior. Often these rules include certain deeply held assumptions about what a man or woman is like. Breaking these rules is highly traumatic, and the confessional voice is a good way to explore this dilemma.

Getting this and other important realizations on paper not only affirms your identity, it clears the way for better communication, improved relationships, and increased self-knowledge. As your personal knowledge grows, it can become the basis for yet another autobiographical voice: the memoir.

The Memoir

The memoir is a record of a specific event compiled from firsthand experience. A good way to use this form is to write about your coming of age. Many people have written coming-of-age memoirs, including Anaïs Nin and Isak Dinesen. So did Helen Keller, whose autobiography, *The Story of My Life*, was first published in a memoir mag-

---

"When you have something to say, to express any form of submission becomes unbearable in the long run. You have to have the courage of your vocation and the courage to live by that vocation."

—PABLO PICASSO, ARTIST

---

azine in 1903. Likewise, Maya Angelou's *I Know Why the Caged Bird Sings* was a memoir that chronicled her life into her early teens.

Angelou also kept a location memoir called *All God's Children Need Traveling Shoes,* which was about her life in Ghana, where she lived for four years. Like Angelou, you, too, might wish to write a location memoir because it can help you interpret new experiences, capture memories, and bring significance to a particular place. The location memoir can also help you reconcile yourself if you're in conflict with your surroundings.

To begin working in this voice, choose a location, then ask yourself what makes this place significant for you. Explore the path that brought you to this place, what gifts this location holds for you, and how this place enhances your senses.

You may also want to use your senses to write an occupational or vocational memoir. If you are an artist, an occupational memoir might be a record of a specific project. It can cover the birth of a particular idea, how you nurtured the idea along, the results, and how those results were perceived by others. The occupational memoir is a good way to measure your professional growth because you can go back to it over the years to assess your progress and glean additional nuggets of inspiration.

You can also use the occupational memoir in a corporate or business setting to track similar issues and realize similar benefits. For instance, perhaps speaking in meetings makes you nervous. By keeping an occupational memoir that includes records of the meetings, your efforts to improve your speaking habits, and the results, the occupational memoir helps you make progress. It can identify your fears, help you learn from those fears, and increase your confidence.

As you can see, the memoir is a very flexible form of the autobiographic voice. Besides coming of age, location, and occupation, you can use it to focus on spirituality, personal philosophy, ecology, politics, society, group life, and an almost limitless number of topics. Regardless of the subject you choose, just remember that the memoir is an autobiographical account with a clearly identified theme. It is at its most dynamic when you include conflict or pairs of opposites to drive your writing forward.

Voices from Fairy Tales

"Once upon a time . . ." Since time immemorial, those words have driven many a powerful story forward. They can do the same for you if you write in the voice of the fairy tale.

A fairy-tale voice can help you capture an incident that seems dreamlike, such as a romance, and get it down on paper so you can examine it more closely. The fairy-tale voice can also support you by taking something grimly realistic, like an accident or emotional trauma, and providing a gentler, more palatable way to explore it. In addition, the fairy tale can aid you in defining the roles of the players in your story: who's the royal princess, the charming prince, the evil witch or warlock, and so on.

To begin writing your story in the fairy-tale voice, pick a time and a situation from childhood. Focus on a desire you pursued or knowledge that changed you. Then open your journal and start with those classic words "Once upon a time there was a little boy or girl who . . ."

Next, advance the fairy tale chronologically and write "Once upon a time there was a man or woman who . . ." Try to write one to two pages about how you grew, what changed, or how the fairy tale had a different ending from what you expected. Use this knowledge to write a letter to a real or imaginary grandchild

Example of a Fairy Tale

"Once there was a little girl who wanted to be an actress because they had beautiful clothes, traveled, and were independent. . . . She asked for dance lessons . . . tried out for plays . . . read actress autobiographies. . . . She graduated from college in three years and then went to acting school in New York where she fell in love with an actor and focused her energy on his career. . . . .She struggled . . . was not happy, got divorced . . . advanced in her career but was lonely . . . so she began a search for her true self. . . . When she reviewed her fairy tale and her pivotal events in her writer's group, her desire line was clear, it was work. Now she accepts that her relationships do not have to be romantic to be life-sustaining and she has remained true to her most important desire—work."

An actress and member of a Chicago writer's group wrote on creating her own fairy tale.

describing the most important insight or wisdom you gained from the fairy tale. Finally, compare the fairy tale to the letter. Do both pieces of writing convey the same insight? If not, what is the insight in the story? The letter? Would another story from your life have more meaning? Whatever the case, writes Tristine Ranier, remember to select a moment in life when you glimpsed your humanity and then work backward or forward from there to create a fairy tale filled with poignancy and power.

Whether it's a fairy tale, a memoir, a confession, or a full autobiography, there are many ways to verbalize the story of your life. Here are a few more suggestions:

* Write autobiographic short stories. Think of these as rings of a tree. One ring might represent childhood, another adolescence, and so on. Although they might seem quite separate, when you put these rings together they tell a complete life story.

* Divide your life by pivotal events. Start with a list of the events, then create a second list. The second list should be things you wanted out of life, that is, the desires that preceded your experiences. Blend the two lists together to

see the relationship between your desires and your actions. Be sure to note any desires you may have left out.

- Write your story as a quest with yourself as the hero or heroine. Begin with your goal. End with whether your goal was achieved and the wisdom you attained. What happened in between the goal and the attainment of wisdom is your autobiographic story.

- Think of your autobiography as a quilt. At first, the individual pieces— your experiences—may not seem related, but put them all together and you gain a cohesive whole.

An Acting Exercise to Help You Find a Voice

Shelly Carlson, actress, well-known Chicago voice teacher and president of Caarlsson Productions, suggests the following acting exercise to help you find your voice.

1. Choose a well-known character from a play, a novel, or fairy tale. Avoid TV characters as they tend to lack depth.

2. Now spend an entire day as your character. Get out of bed like your character, bathe like your character, have what he or she would have for breakfast, speak as your character would speak, read aloud as your character would read, and so on. Carlson also recommends using props the way your character would use them. For instance, would your character use a fountain pen or a computer, drink cocoa made from scratch or in the microwave, and so on.

3. Review yourself from head to toe. If you are in character, you will have a distinct voice and a different way of using your body. You may speak and move more sensually, have a softer tone or touch, approach your world with more awareness.

4. Next, write in your journal in your character's voice. This can be a note, a letter, memoir, or any autobiographic format as long as it's in your character's voice.

5. Now think about your own voice, your tone and intent, the way you use words. Use your heightened awareness from this exercise to think of yourself as a true-life character, says Carlson, and you will move a step closer to writing your authentic voice.

"Perhaps this is the strongest pleasure known to me . . . the rapture I get when in writing I seem to be discovering what belongs to what; making a scene come right; making a character come together . . . behind the cotton wool [of daily life] is hidden a pattern; that we—I mean all human beings—are connected with this; that the whole world is a work of art."

—VIRGINIA WOOLF FROM *A SKETCH OF THE PAST*

FOUND IN HER UNPUBLISHED AUTOBIOGRAPHICAL WRITINGS

◆ Try a hybrid autobiography that combines autobiographic writing with something else you love. For instance, M.F.K. Fisher combined memoirs and cookbooks. You can do something similar with confessions and automobiles, fairy tales and geography, or anything that strikes you as a good combination and helps you tell your life story.

Perhaps the best thing about autobiographic writing—telling your life story—is that it eschews labels, theories, and analysis, and concentrates on words, your words. Happily those words are not the province of any particular age, race, or socioeconomic class. In fact, the autobiographic journal gives the disenfranchised or rarely heard from a much needed voice. It gives everyone's life meaning because you tell your story from your perspective, and this alone makes your experience worthy of contemplation and expression. There's another advantage to autobiographical writing as well.

Many writers feel the patterns in the autobiographic journal reveal the hand of a Higher Power or express the spiritual mystery in the shape and form of their individual lives. You, too, might discover this as you write in an autobiographic voice.

The Voice of Humankind

A voice that addresses humankind in general often focuses on points of morality, government policy, poverty, prejudice, and disease. In *At a Journal Workshop*, Ira Progoff noted "Our dialogue with Society can . . . enable us to maintain a continuing relationship with the political events of our time. We may be in dialogue with our country, with its leaders, and with the general issues that are at the fore of discussion. At times of political turbulence, it becomes especially important to have an instrument like the journal workbook to clarify our personal role in the events taking place."

Many famous public documents and essays started life as journal entries addressed to the world at large. Ralph Waldo Emerson, Henry David Thoreau, Thomas Paine, Michel de Montaigne, Blaise Pascal, Denis Diderot, Jean-Jacques Rousseau, Immanuel Kant, Friedrich von Schiller, Johann Wolfgang von Goethe, Jonathan Swift, Samuel Pepys, Thomas Aquinas, and others expressed in their journals the deep desire to alter situations and work for change. Eventually this desire led some of these journal writers to seek a more public forum through newspapers and magazines, or, in the case of those writing today, through broadcast media or the Internet.

Gore Vidal, winner of a National Book Award for *United States: Essays 1952–1992*, carries on this time-honored tradition of addressing humankind with chronicles of the American political and moral climate, as when he wrote "every now and then, usually

Creating a Visual Guide to Help You Address Humankind

A Visual Guide is an actual picture of a reality you're trying to achieve. It helps form a clear image of your vision for humankind so you can bring energy and actualization to this goal. The Visual Guide is a powerful nonverbal way to collect your thoughts and translate those thoughts into words in your journal. Just follow these steps.

1. Decide on your message to humankind.

2. Make a collage using images that visualize your message. These can be pictures or words cut from magazines, books, cards, photos, drawings, or paintings. If you wish, include yourself in the pictures. Just be sure to show the situation at its ideal level.

3. Translate the image into words in your journal.

4. If you choose, share your words and your Visual Guide with humankind.

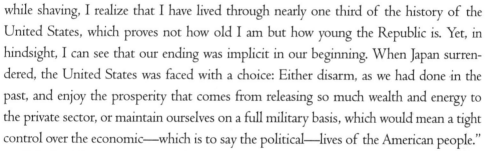

The Voice of Historical Perspective

The power of writing about your life and times so that future generations gain a sense of historical perspective is amply demonstrated in Ken Burns's acclaimed television documentaries *The Civil War, Brooklyn Bridge, Baseball, Thomas Jefferson,* and *Frank Lloyd Wright.* The journal excerpts, diaries, and letters that formed the foundation for these programs expressed the universality of human experience through individual voices.

You, too, can use your individual voice to help future generations understand historical perspective. Your unique point of view and interpretation of the events around you, coupled with accurate names, dates, descriptions, and references, can help future generations understand your era as you saw it. You can write about this from a very personal level, perhaps addressing a future grandchild, or from a broader perspective that addresses all of humankind.

while shaving, I realize that I have lived through nearly one third of the history of the United States, which proves not how old I am but how young the Republic is. Yet, in hindsight, I can see that our ending was implicit in our beginning. When Japan surrendered, the United States was faced with a choice: Either disarm, as we had done in the past, and enjoy the prosperity that comes from releasing so much wealth and energy to the private sector, or maintain ourselves on a full military basis, which would mean a tight control over the economic—which is to say the political—lives of the American people."

Like Vidal, you can write to humankind. While it is not necessary for you to print or broadcast your journal entries unless you wish to do so, you can address any topic you care enough to write about and express how it applies to the general population. Interestingly enough, almost every topic will apply in some way. Why?

Eric Maisel, author of *Deep Writing,* explains that "each of us is a human being. Each of us recapitulates human nature in a particular way. Each of us is a product of heredity and environment. Each of us is troubled and challenged in multiple ways. Each of us has appetites, dreams, ambitions, doubts, anxieties, love, prejudices, and depressions." These similarities provide the links between your journal and humankind.

Your personal interpretation, rationale, and the passion with which you infuse your entries will allow you to organize your thoughts, decide if you wish to take your concerns public, and express how you might persuade others to support your point of view. One way to do this is to imagine something of great value, something you want very much. This can be the righting of a social wrong, a position, an honor—anything you care deeply about. Now imagine yourself mounting a campaign to achieve this goal. Muster all your firepower, whether it is political influence, public opinion, or verbal salvos. Whatever the means, envision yourself battling as long and hard as necessary to reach your objective.

If you feel resistance to writing about such a no-holds-barred assault, remember that this is just a daydream, not reality, and then proceed. When you have attained your goal in writing, enjoy it and process your feelings of success. Describe the experience in your journal and see if you want to translate your daydream into reality for yourself or for humankind.

Writing in a Spiritual Voice

The voice you use to write spiritual entries varies. You might express yourself in respectful prayers or meditations, or you might write a dialogue between yourself and the Divine Power. You also might find yourself complaining or making belligerent demands, but if you do, don't worry. You're in the good company of people like Latin scholar St. Jerome (A.D. 340–420), who demanded to know "why did I come from the womb, to see sorrow and pain, and to end my days in shame?"

If this sounds familiar, says the prophet Jeremiah, remember that anger, frustration, and railing against the Supreme Being are clear expressions of your passion for spirituality and your desire to understand. In fact, Jeremiah describes this very voice as part of the aspirant's path when he writes "you are chosen, you resist, you resort to rage and bitterness and, finally you succumb to the god who has given you your identity in the first place." These words of Jeremiah assure you that far from being disrespectful, a quarrelsome voice has spiritual dimensions when it's used in a quest for divine understanding.

There are other voices you can use for divine understanding too. Hildegard of Bingen was a twelfth-century abbess who lived in a convent with a liturgical tradition. As part of this tradition, Hildegard read scriptures, prayed, and recorded her responses in a spiritual journal.

Writing about her experiences allowed Hildegard to see her spiritual progress both literally and figuratively as when she described this revelation: "When I was forty-two years and seven months old, a burning light of tremendous brightness coming from heaven poured into my entire mind like a flame that does not burn but enkindles. It enflamed my entire heart. All at once I was able to taste of the understanding of books, the Psalter, the Evangelists, and the books of the Old and New Testaments."

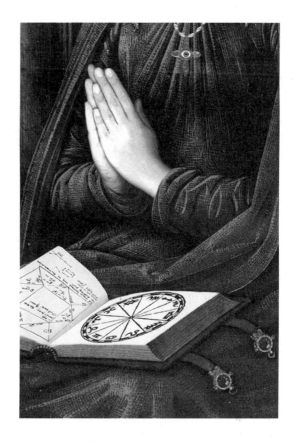

(fragment) *Astrology Reader,* © Lois Guarino, 1997, courtesy of Robert Mann Gallery, NYC

You, too, can find understanding when you write in a spiritual voice, and that voice can follow any number of traditions. You might copy Islamic prayers and chants in your journal or Buddhist meditations that help you seek God within. You might travel the Hindu path, using your journal to chart efforts to enter the illusory world and achieve unity with a Higher Power. If you choose a Native American tradition, your journal can incorporate drawings that trace the flight of the eagle, the divine messenger who moves between this world and the world of the Creators. Regardless of the dialect you choose, your spiritual voice will ask why and how. It will seek to gain and share knowledge. Ultimately the answers will come.

You are more likely to find these answers when you write about spiritual research and practices, divine experiences and revelations. It may also be helpful to copy read-

Preparation for Working in a Spiritual Voice

Bhante Y. Wimala is a Buddhist monk from Sri Lanka and an Omega meditation faculty member. He offers the following suggestions to cultivate awareness of the choices you make. You may find them helpful as you choose a spiritual voice for your journal:

+ On rising every morning, make a conscious choice to experience the day's blessings.

+ Choose acceptance over resistance when people or things do not turn out as expected.

+ In negative situations, make a conscious choice to respond with calmness and self-assurance.

+ Choose kindness toward yourself and others.

ings and affirmations that clarify and strengthen your spiritual path. This is invaluable when your path changes, as Trappist monk Thomas Merton attested.

Merton published *Secular Journal* in 1959. It is his account of the years 1939 to 1941, before his entrance into the monastery. He wrote that the journal explores "the essential incommunicability of the highest form of religious experience" and his attempts to choose between a monastic life and a more socially involved one at Friendship House, a Catholic mission in Harlem.

Merton's journal records this struggle and his spiritual movement from an active life to a contemplative one. The road was not easy, and Merton was among the first Americans to write honestly and lucidly about this conflict. He continued to publish a book each decade based on some aspect of his religious journals and his spiritual voice.

Likewise, Thomas Moore, professor of religion, psychology, and a former member of a monastic order, says "...spiritual writing...in journals...is not just a way to communicate or to keep a record; primarily it's a form of contemplation." In other words, your journal is a source of spirit first and foremost. For this reason, you should approach your entries with reverence and remember that your spiritual voice is sacred. Writing in this sacred voice imbues your writing with its own deep mystery and makes your journal a book of wisdom in the great tradition of other holy books. Indeed, says Moore, "many of our personal problems stem from the loss of individuality, expressiveness, intimacy, and power; and potent, spell-binding language can help us keep and restore those important qualities." It can also lead you to your spiritual home.

Whether you use your journal to reach your spiritual home or to describe your autobiographic one, to speak like an adult or a child, to address humankind or speak from a historical perspective, these voices are all part of you, who you are, who you were, and who you have the potential to become. As you change and grow in different directions over the years, even more voices will speak up, wanting to be heard and recorded in your journal. When you pair them to a topic and an approach, you not only preserve them, you create a dialogue for life.

TO LEARN MORE ABOUT VOICE, READ:

Allione, Tsultrim. *Women of Wisdom* (London: Routledge & Kegan Paul, 1984).

Blume, Judy. *Tales of a Fourth Grade Nothing* (New York: E. P. Dutton, 1972).

Mallon, Thomas. *A Book of One's Own* (St. Paul, Minn.: Hungry Mind Press, 1986).

Norris, Kathleen. *The Cloister Walk* (New York: Riverhead Books, 1996).

Ranier, Tristine. *Your Life as Story: Discovering the New Autobiography* (Garden City, N.Y.: Tarcher/Putnam, 1988).

Russell, Bertrand. *Why I Am Not a Christian* (New York: Simon and Schuster, 1957).

Schiwy, Marlene. *A Voice of Her Own: Women and the Journal-Writing Journey* (New York: Simon and Schuster, 1996).

Vidal, Gore. *At Home, Essays, 1982–1988* (New York: Random House, 1988).

Wimala, Bhante Y. *Lessons of the Lotus: Practical Spiritual Teachings of a Traveling Buddhist Monk* (New York: Bantam Books, 1997).

FOR GOOD EXAMPLES OF WRITING TO HUMANKIND, TRY:

French, Marilyn. *Beyond Power* (New York: Ballantine, 1985).

Laing, R. D. *The Politics of Experience* (New York: Ballantine, 1967).

Lewis, C. S. *Mere Christianity* (New York: Macmillan, 1945).

Singer, June. *Androgyny: Toward a New Theory of Sexuality* (Garden City, N.Y.: Figo Press, 1987).

FOR RESOURCES ON THE SPIRITUAL VOICE, READ:

Communion: Contemporary Writers Reveal the Bible in Their Lives (New York: Anchor Books, 1996).

Moore, Thomas. *The Re-Enchantment of Everyday Life* (New York: Harper Collins, 1996).

Norris, Kathleen. *The Cloister Walk* (New York: Riverhead Books, 1996).

Weiner, Herbert. *9/1/2 Mystics: The Kabbala Today* (New York: Macmillan, 1969).

For good examples of a wide range of journal "voices" in online journals, visit "Tracing: Journal of Daily Thoughts and Events" at www.ounce.com/links.html

7

Learning from Your Journal

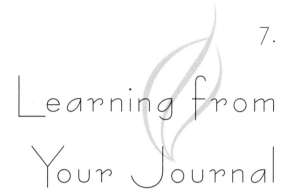

Writing a journal can be instructive, but analyzing what you've written—with some distance and a new perspective—can help you learn even more. Study and analysis can reveal deeper meanings, promote self-understanding, and help you grow, and that is the whole point. As British poet laureate C. Day Lewis, author of *The Poetic Image*, stated "we do not write in order to be understood, we write in order to understand."

To support this understanding, it's a good idea to review past journal entries. Doing so probably is most valuable when you experience something that changes your life or when you want to reconnect with an emotion related to your original writing. After all, the best way to appreciate change is to understand where you've been and compare it to where you are. Past journal entries can help in this regard, particularly if you are evaluating whether the current change is a direction you want to go. Likewise, using your journal to reconnect with a particular feeling can help you measure your emotional maturity, revitalize a memory, or recapture a passion to use in some creative way.

Start by reserving quiet, uninterrupted time just for you. After you eliminate all possible distractions, take a moment to clear your thoughts so you can approach your journal in a nonjudgmental way. This is important because an open mind leaves you receptive to new lessons and unexpected finds. Once you're in this state, begin slowly rereading your journal entries.

Take the time to absorb your words and accept their meaning with compassion, just as you would while reading a letter from an old friend. As you read, track the dominant emotions expressed in your writing. For example, do you often write about frustration? Are love, joy, or anger consistently expressed?

These patterns are the key to learning from your journal. You can look for emotional repetition, universal truths that keep resurfacing, or questions that come up again and again. Seeing evidence of these and other cycles may promote new energy, growth, and a fresh point of view. This knowledge can also help you rebuild your personal infrastructure and use your entries to support the person you want to become.

One way to begin this process is by looking at categories. What is the topic you write about most often? Is it your family or intimate relationship? Work or hobbies? Your health? Perhaps your entries focus more on one area than you realized. If this is a surprise to you, you might want to give this part of your life more conscious attention. Maybe this category represents a decision you must make in order to move ahead; or maybe it's a source of great joy for you and is something you should consider as a full-time profession, life philosophy, or gift of grace you can share with others.

Just as you can learn a great deal from the categories you do write about, you can learn a great deal from the categories you don't write about. Take a close look at what's missing from your journal. Are you practicing self-censorship? Leaving something out of your entries because you're afraid of hurting someone else or are unwilling or unable to face an issue yourself? If so, try making a list of your omissions and study it for patterns. Use the list to move toward self-acceptance or to consider alternatives. This process can increase your self-compassion, clarify your goals, and help you direct both your life energy and your future journal entries in a purposeful way.

To reinforce these benefits, include the list as one of your journal entries and revisit it at appropriate intervals. This is particularly important if self-censorship is a continuing concern. If it is, you may want to keep two journals, one that is uncensored and just for you and one that you edit to share with others. Just remember, even if you keep a private journal, self-censorship might still creep into your writing. If it does, ask yourself what lesson there is in this. If the self-censorship is sending you a message, write about it. Periodic checks can build your awareness and help you make progress with this and other issues.

In fact, as you review your entries you might be pleasantly surprised by your perceptions, willpower, writing ability, coping mechanisms, and belief in yourself. Evidence of these positive patterns is right on the page. When you see them, these qualities can reinforce your self-esteem and build your sense of accomplishment. This is a marvelous gift your journal entries provide.

Your journal can also give you the gift of spirituality. By studying your entries, you may see moments of Divine inspiration, blessings in your everyday life, and confirmation of your calling. Analyzing your journal for the presence of spirit is also a great tool for working through depression and helping you cope with the setbacks we all experience in life.

Analyzing Setbacks and Your Reaction to Change

As you analyze setbacks, it's important to identify who or what robs you of power and energy. Then you need to learn from this adversity and increase your ability to cope. Your journal can help with the following steps.

First, writes Dr. Caroline Myss, a prominent leader in holistic consciousness, use your journal to do an energy audit of the people, experiences, and information you allow into your life. In other words, who or what is draining you? Is this drain emotional or physical? Financial or spiritual? How long do the effects last?

Study this in your journal, then create a list of affirmations and action steps that can help you preserve your energy. For instance, does Aunt Martha always call with bad news? If you identify her conversations as an energy drain, you have several options. Maybe you could direct the conversation in a more positive way, limit the time you're willing to spend talking about negative things, or take her calls only when you really feel up to it. You could also work to accept Aunt Martha as she is and not be flustered by her negativity.

Myss notes this process takes time, attention, and daily practice, but your journal can ease the way. It can help you discover solutions, solutions that are more likely to

> "In most lives insight has been accidental. We wait for it as primitive man awaited lightning for a fire. But making mental connections is our most crucial learning tool, the essence of human intelligence; to forge links; to go beyond the given; to see patterns, relationship; context."
>
> —MARILYN FERGUSON, *THE AQUARIAN CONSPIRACY*

succeed if you keep them simple. This is where your entries come in handy. You can use them to brainstorm, evaluate options, track results, build your patience, and strive for balance.

"Remind yourself that life is to learn to balance the energies of body and soul, of thought and action, of physical and mental power," explains Myss. To create that balance, you must try to accept the fact that any life circumstance can change in the blink of an eye. When this happens, remember that the important thing is to be true to yourself and to seek happiness from within. This is easier if you acknowledge that change is constant.

With that in mind, look at your journal entries. Highlight or underline passages that illustrate your reactions to change. Do they show that you found change easy or hard to accept? Is it a repeating pattern? Despite changing circumstances, were you true to yourself? Were you your own source of happiness and contentment? How does your journal reflect this? What lessons do you see in your response to change?

As you analyze these issues in your journal, remember to practice forgiveness toward yourself and others. Also remember that positive energy is more effective than negative energy. Applying these principles to your life will improve your ability to cope with change, help you move forward, and live more fully in the moment.

Analyzing Your Journal by Images

According to Shelly Carlson, actress, voice teacher, and originator of the popular course "Speaking and Writing the Way People Think," another way to learn from your journal is to analyze the images you see in your words. Analyzing by imagery means realizing that not all your words have equal weight.

A good way to become familiar with this technique is to open up a book of fairy tales and select a descriptive phrase three to six words in length. Silently repeat the phrase to yourself, then study the way your mind interprets it. What you will find is that you think in images and you draw these images from the entire phrase, not from single words. For instance, with the phrase "a little red house," you don't see "a," followed by a vision of "little," followed by "red," followed by "house." Instead, your mind puts the individual words together to form a bigger picture.

With this awareness in mind, go to your journal and select one page. Place parentheses around all the images you find. You will discover that specific images have specific meanings and associations as they resurface in your entries. This image repetition is a useful shorthand system for accessing your emotional trends. In fact, if you record these patterns in an Image Index, you will have a veritable pictogram that can guide you in analyzing your journal and understanding who you are.

To create an Image Index, make a simple chart that catalogs your visual symbols. At the top of the page insert these four headings running left to right: Image, Frequency, Life Experience, Dominant Emotion.

Under Image, write a description or draw a picture of the visual symbol. Don't worry if your drawing is primitive. Just get a sense of what your image looks like. Now move to Frequency. How often does the image appear in your entries? Daily? Weekly? Only in moments of deep emotion? Note it on your chart. Next, go to Life Experiences. What's happening in your life when this image appears? Are the same circumstances present whenever you write about this image? Finally, move to Dominant Emotion. Ask yourself what feeling you associate with the image. Is the same emotion present every time the symbol appears in your entries?

Chart your images over a period of months. Eventually they will reveal patterns

---

". . . the image is as real as a table or the galaxies. The image matters. Matters as much as anything matters. The image is the prima materia. To respect it, work with it, live with it, act upon it, finally to live it is the very core of a creative life."

—DEENA METZGER

Strengthening Your Imagery Through Language Tools

This exercise will help you practice your skill with literary tools and expand your capacity for writing powerful images in your journal.

◆ Look at a scene for thirty to sixty seconds.

◆ Listen to the way your mind describes it. If you think "what a pretty sky," try to be more specific, as in "what a painterly spring sky with its wisps of clouds and flocks of geese."

◆ Insert your emotional response to the scene: "What a great day to be alive."

◆ Insert a color. Don't make it a "nice sky"; call it "a robin's egg blue sky with clouds the color of vanilla frosting."

◆ Now use assonance to describe the scene: "The sky was dry."

◆ Try it again using alliteration, as in "The sky was simply spectacular."

◆ Think of the scene in onomatopoeia, "The sun slipped beneath the horizon."

◆ Finally, use simile—"The sky was as gold as honey"—and metaphor—"When the sun sank, it dripped honey gold light on the corn" to describe what you see.

that help you visualize goals, dreams, positive and negative associations, and life lessons. They also provide the basis for a dictionary of symbols with which to analyze your journal.

Since imagery requires extensive work with language, you may want to increase your linguistic abilities. Start by asking yourself if you use single words where a phrase would be more specific, evocative, and interesting. If so, take some of these words and turn them into phrases that create stronger, more meaningful pictures. For instance, instead of writing "I'm cold" write "I was so cold my soul turned blue," or "It was so cold my tongue stuck to the enamel of my teeth."

You can also enlarge your vocabulary with the following technique. Buy an inexpensive paperback dictionary and tear out one page at a time. Attach it to your bathroom mirror so you can learn a new word whenever you brush your teeth. Then use these new words to write full descriptions rather than qualifiers. For example, instead of writing "It was pretty painful" or "It really hurt," try "It stung like a thousand lashes." Another idea is to use more specific words in place of your usual vocabulary. To do this, look up one of your words in a thesaurus, then write down all the other options on a card. Attach the card to your bathroom mirror and learn a new option every day.

If you are using your journal to improve your writing skills, you can also apply certain advanced language devices to increase the power of your word images, such as *assonance.* Assonance is a strong repeating vowel sound, as in p<u>a</u>le and br<u>a</u>ve; *alliteration,* the repetition of a consonant sound as in <u>d</u>eep, <u>d</u>ark, <u>d</u>itch; *onomatopoeia,* a word that sounds like what it means, as in a "silky, slinky, slip of a dress"; *simile,* a comparison using the words *like* or *as;* or *metaphor,* a comparison that attributes a particular quality to a subject, usually a quality that is not literally applicable, such as "nerves of steel" or "an icy glance." Just remember that it's your choice whether to use these language tools; with or without them, your authentic voice will come through.

Besides language techniques, there are other ways to make your images more dynamic. One is with cadence and the rhythmic flow of your words as in "the rat-a-tat-tat of his quick questions." Color is helpful too, both as a physical and emotional adjective like "blood red" or "sad yellow." Finally, threading, which is the meaningful repetition of an image throughout your entries, can make your writing come alive.

What else can you do to strengthen your imagery? Try reading good literature and poetry. Examples from poetry are particularly helpful if you tend to overwrite and obscure the important image. In addition, you can join a book group or chat room to practice your writing skills; study grammar; look at a painting or sculpture and describe your response using the preceding techniques; or read your entries into a tape recorder, then play them back to become aware of overused words or phrases and substitutions you can make.

As your language skills grow and you are able to express yourself more vividly, your imagery will become increasingly potent. You will reduce self-censorship and develop more accurate, detailed descriptions of your experiences. These details provide a greater level of information with which to analyze your feelings and life direction and become acquainted with who you are.

Using Lists to Analyze Your Journal

Lists are a means of visual organization, a way of distilling your thoughts and words to their most powerful essence. By recombining your entries into lists, you can see patterns in your experience and pave the way for behavior changes.

Consultant and motivational speaker Joyce Chapman suggests in her book that you start with a list of things you do well. Cull through your journal entries and find everything that fits this description. Then put these items in a list using short, bullet-point descriptions. When you're finished, you have a handy tool that tracks your abilities and reinforces your self-confidence whenever you're feeling low.

Likewise, a list of things you love or that make you feel fulfilled can help when life seems empty; a list of your good qualities and positive experiences can balance things out when your ego has taken a blow; and a list of people you like being with and who like being with you can help when you feel lonely. Other lists are useful too.

Listing the ways you are like your parents can give you a sense of continuity or, on the opposite end of the spectrum, help you analyze traditional viewpoints that no longer serve you well. A list of excuses or times you've been wrong can be an excellent tool for rebuilding your character. Chapman also suggests using lists to analyze the times you've been acknowledged, moments you were right, gains, losses, and celebrations. In fact, almost any journal entry can be the basis of a list and practically any list can become a journal entry if you use it to gain insight and change your behavior.

Analyzing Your Journal by Word Clusters

Word clusters are groups of words that can be associated with either your logical, practical self or your intuitive, creative self. According to university professor and creative writing consultant Lusser Gabriele Rico, your logical self edits, refines, and rewrites what you've produced. By contrast, your intuitive self lets you experiment, apply your imagination, and follow your instincts. By working with word clusters, you can use your journal to learn about the relationship between these two sides of your brain.

To start, choose one word from your journal and write it on a fresh page. Circle it, then rapidly write down any connecting words that occur to you. Circle each connecting word, then let your thoughts radiate out in any direction you choose to find more new words. Write them down. Use a line to connect each new word to the preceding circle. A variation on this method is to look in your journal and relate key words from different sentences. You can either pull these words out individually and apply the cluster method or simply circle clusters of words that appear together in your entries.

Rico states that far from being random, word clusters reveal deep associations that show you how your emotions, your intellect, and your spirit are organized. Seeing how your thoughts are connected can clarify relationships, promote insights, boost self-awareness, and help you break the bonds of self-censorship. Ultimately, this helps you use your inner eye to direct your writing and your life.

Using Your Journal to Learn About Your Dreams

Dreams are a rich resource for your outer life and your inner work. Whether that work is physical, emotional, spiritual, or creative, you can benefit from keeping a journal where you preserve your dreams and analyze them on a regular basis. While you can include this writing in your daily entries, you might want to keep it in a separate place since you should record your dreams as soon as possible and this is likely to happen late at night or in the wee hours of the morning. Both time slots are excellent reasons to keep your journal by your bed and, if you're not alone, to write in pen instead of pencil. The sound of a pencil scratching across paper can seem annoying in the quiet of night. So can turning on the overhead light, so use a small reading light or pen light instead.

With your tools in place, you're set to record your dreams. Write them down while they are still fresh in your memory and include as much detail and richness as possible. Of course, you can do this only if you remember what you dreamed about, so here's a way to improve your memory. When you wake up, lie quietly with your eyes closed. Pay careful attention to anything you remember from last night's sleep, no matter how small. You might remember only an image, a sound, an emotion, or a physical sensation; that's okay. Focus on this memory but don't work too hard at it since it's important for you to stay relaxed and open-minded. See if anything else comes to mind, then write down everything you recall in your dream journal. Once you begin to write, other impressions or the full dream may follow. If it doesn't, don't worry.

You don't need to remember every dream you've ever had in order to gain insight into their meanings. Dream information is persistent. If you miss the point the first time around, your dreams will give you a second chance by presenting the same information in another way. Just be patient, give yourself time, and remain receptive. By consistently trying to remember your dreams, you establish a routine that will enhance your memory. In addition, your desire to remember will help you focus.

If you try this and, after several weeks, still have trouble remembering your dreams, use this simple technique. As you fall asleep, tell yourself over and over that you *will* remember your dreams. Although it sounds simple and may not work right away, this affirmation is highly effective and eventually will lead to greater dream recall.

Just tell yourself that you will wake up after each dream prepared to write it down,

Creating a Memory Fragment Worksheet to Use with Your Dreams

To help you remember dream fragments that occur throughout the day, take a sheet of paper and across the top write Date, Place, and Memory/Other Information. Use the sheet to record any spontaneous memories that flash across your mind, then use this information to help you record and analyze dreams in your journal. Finally, insert the completed memory fragment worksheets in your journal for safekeeping.

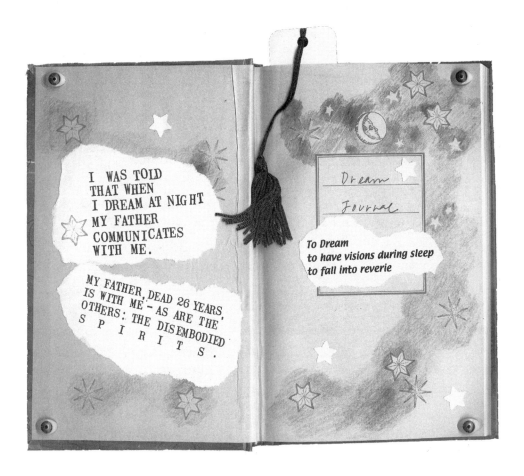

I WAS TOLD
THAT WHEN
I DREAM AT NIGHT
MY FATHER
COMMUNICATES
WITH ME.

MY FATHER, DEAD 26 YEARS,
IS WITH ME - AS ARE THE
OTHERS: THE DISEMBODIED
S P I R I T S.

Dream
Journal

To Dream
to have visions during sleep
to fall into reverie

Inside cover of a dream journal
from the journal collection of the author

and do this regardless of the hour. Why? If you don't record your dreams immediately, they might just slip away. This is more likely to happen if your normal sleeping and waking patterns are interrupted by the sound of the alarm, noise in your room, or someone shaking you awake.

Fortunately, lost memories can return at a later time. You probably remember moments in the past when a dream fragment seemed to appear out of nowhere. In all likelihood, a word, a color, or a sound stimulated your memory and the whole dream came flooding back. Many times this happens when you're involved in some elementary task and your mind is free to wander. Even though you can't plan for these moments, you need to acknowledge them when they occur. Don't repress or dismiss them; instead, be receptive to this type of recollection and write it down in your journal. That way you can study what provoked the memory and how it relates to your dream.

Sometimes you don't need these memory assists. In fact, often, upon waking, you may have a very clear recollection of your dream. To help you retain it, keep your eyes closed and try to run through the dream visually, like a movie played on fast speed in your head. This should help you remember all the vivid details that you might otherwise forget. When you've gone through the dream at least once, write it down in your journal. Include the smallest fragments or seemingly insignificant details and how you feel about the dream. Use these emotions to give your dream a title. The title usually highlights the most significant aspect of your dream and is an excellent clue to what type of dream it is.

While your dream world is unique, most dreams fall into certain categories, and figuring out where your dream fits is a good way to grasp its meaning. You might dream about current experiences or have emotional overspill dreams that express the anxieties of your day. Illness, injury, or other physical factors can affect the content of your dreams, or dreams might have a strong moral-of-the-story element. You might have an inspirational dream that plants fertile ideas for self-expression and creative work. There are also precognitive dreams that predict future events and spiritual dreams of transformation. Highly visual, nonverbal dreams can provide guidance while problem-solving dreams may give you insights into troubling life issues. In short, there are as many types of dreams as there are people, and writing about them helps you understand what you've experienced.

One way to see if you're dreaming about daily events is to write Day Notes in your journal. Before you fall asleep, write down anything you consider to be important about your day, including significant events in your personal and professional life and any emotions associated with them. You should also note how you feel physically. Be sure to use only the highlights of your day, things you would consider interesting enough to reread several months down the line. After you record your dreams, compare them to your Day Notes and see if the two have anything in common. Perhaps your dreams are trying to give you a message about something or trying to help you solve a problem you encountered during the day.

Questions to Ask in Your Analysis of Dreams

As you work to decipher your dreams, these points may help to shed some light. Write the answers in your journal.

+ What was at work in your dream?

+ How easy or difficult was it to remember your dream?

+ What do you face in the day ahead?

+ List any symbols in your dream.

+ Do these symbols have universal meaning? Personal meaning?

+ What is the theme of your dream?

+ Draw or otherwise visually interpret your dream.

If you would like this kind of assistance, use your journal to describe the problem. Write down as many pertinent facts or questions as you can think of, then read them over before going to sleep. As you drift off, ask your dreams for answers. Just making this suggestion to yourself can influence the content of your dreams and how you interpret them the next day, and these interpretations are valuable tools.

Using your journal to record the content, meaning, and titles of your dreams provides you with an excellent reference by which to measure future dreams and states of mind. In addition, by preserving them on paper, you can access what you've dreamed in the past and build your own system of dream symbols. Symbols are things that recur and have deeper meaning. These can be universal symbols, such as those found in art, religion, myth, or specific cultures, or they can be images, words, actions, or characters that are significant only to you. Fortunately, you don't have to know what these symbols mean, only that they're important.

Eventually, through additional dreams and the journal-writing experience, the meaning of these symbols will come through. Sometimes that meaning may relate to conditions outside your dream world. For instance, the sound of a bell in your dream

"I met a stranger sitting at a small table in a café. He was a middle-aged man with a very gentle manner. We began talking and I knew instantly that I was able to be quite open and trusting with him. We talked about his life. He was in the theater. He promised to tell me about his next production so that I could see him perform. I wrote my address on a page of my spiral notebook and left, forgetting the pad with him. The next day, the pad arrived with a page done by him. There were also several fanciful writings and drawings on random pages. It occurred to me that it was a forum for our communication—a dream book—and so I set about making a cover for the book. I constructed a collage which covered the original binding. In large informal letters I wrote: *The Dream Book, a Collaboration.* I was pleased by both the project and the fact that it was aptly named: the book having originated in the dream of which I was a part at that very moment! I drew a picture, did some writings, and mailed the book back to the man I had met in the café. I hoped that he would know that we would continue to share the book, back and forth, until the dreaming was finished."

—ONE OF THE AUTHOR'S DREAMS THAT INSPIRED A DREAM JOURNAL

might be the alarm clock in your room or a dream of freezing weather might mean you've kicked off the covers. Under other circumstances, these same dream symbols might have totally different meanings, but only you will know for sure. Only you really know what your dreams are about, and you must trust yourself to make this interpretation. Let go of rational, linear thought and go on instinct. Your journal entries can help by giving you a place to work with these revealing questions:

What part of the dream caused you the strongest emotional reaction? What was this reaction and did you feel this way during the day? Does the dream narrative refer back to your Day Notes? Are physical or emotional factors playing a part in your dream? What symbols are present in your dream and what do they mean?

As you work with these questions, you will not only learn about your dreams, you will tap into your inner wisdom and extend your self-knowledge. You will access your subconscious in a tangible way that can improve your insights, your decisions, and your life.

Using Your Journal to Learn About the Connection Between Your Emotional and Physical Health

Many physical and emotional problems are related. Your journal can help you analyze this relationship and use the knowledge to improve your health on both levels. Kary Broffman, R.N., C.H., has a guided imagery and hypnosis practice in Rhinebeck, New York. She sees clients with a range of concerns including stress management, medical issues, and addictive behaviors. Broffman says, "Often people come to me and they don't know how to access their imaginations. I reply that imagery takes practice and remind them that we all use images daily. If we can image or conceive fear and worry—which we all do so well—we can learn how to image anything we want. Hypnosis is utilized to help people make behavioral changes and shift perspectives. I find that prescribing a journal for everyday thoughts, dreams, and life experiences helps my clients to begin to explore the imagery that comes forth as a tool in the healing journey."

One of Broffman's clients came to see her because she was experiencing the disturbing sensation of having her throat close down. "Through our work together," Broffman explains, "it became clear that the actual events of her life were trapped in her body. Twenty years earlier she had been attacked and choked. Although physically she had not been injured, she carried the traumatic experience in her body, specifically in her throat. This caused her daily physical discomfort to the point where she needed medication to ease her symptoms in order to function. The guided imagery and the journal writing helped this woman to see that her physical problems were symbolic of or a metaphor for her life's experiences. Once she explored the experience, she was able to let go and forgive. Her journal entries helped bring the pieces together so that she could see the whole picture. After twenty years of suffering, she is now free of all her symptoms and no longer needs medication."

To use your journal in a similar way, start with Broffman's creative visualization for healing. It works like this. Close your eyes and relax every part of your body. Begin

Debrena Jackson Gandy's Pampering Suggestions

In *Sacred Pampering Principles, An African American Woman's Guide to Self-Care and Inner Renewal*, Debrena Jackson Gandy suggests the following to care for your body and soul:

+ Take a day off from work to pamper yourself. Instead of a sick day, Gandy recommends calling it a day of renewal.

+ Stay home and relax for an entire weekend.

+ Invite a friend over for good conversation. For a change of pace, sit on the floor instead of on the couch or in chairs.

+ Browse through a bookstore and take all the time you want.

+ Go on a nature hike alone.

+ Climb into your pajamas as soon as you get home from work.

+ Have a family member make you breakfast in bed.

at the top of your head and work down to the tips of your toes. Visualize a healing light or wave of energy flowing through your body. When you are relaxed, imagine yourself in a place that is peaceful and safe, where you feel calm and in control.

Now ask for help from your higher self or from another source that you feel provides strength and guidance. Ask a direct question pertaining to an issue in your life. Wait for an answer. The answer may come in the form of a word, voice, picture, or feeling in your body. Don't attempt to interpret it. Just take what comes.

Slowly open your eyes and begin writing about your experience in your journal without editing. If nothing comes forth, don't worry, just continue to practice. Eventually, as time goes by, more information will surface. When it does, continue to write it down. At a certain point, says Broffman, you will have enough information to start putting the pieces together and will recognize the pattern and sources of your feelings.

Besides your life history, you can use emotional issues that are linked with traditional physical ailments to analyze your journal. For example, writes Caroline Myss, Ph.D., problems in your feet or spine may be related to concerns about supporting yourself or your family; sore throats are often associated with conflicts over personal expression and strength of will; and nervous system ailments may be associated with feelings of inadequacy and low self-esteem. Your journal can help you make these connections, determine if you need professional assistance, and if so, what kind.

To aid you in this process, Myss writes that you must first identify the emotional issue that is draining energy from your body and then disconnect from it. Invoke the help of your higher self. Call upon your honesty, integrity, and endurance. Feel the energy of love and compassion fill you, and give this energy to yourself and others. Instead of judging yourself, pay attention to the quality of your thoughts. Focus on self-care and ask for divine guidance to change the patterns set in place by your fears. Ask the spirit to aid you if you feel frightened or confused, then use the experience to weaken your fears, strengthen your soul, and support your physical self.

Try to look at your entries with wonder, analyze them with honesty, and act on them with courage. Supporting your health and well-being is what learning from your journal is all about.

FOR OTHER WAYS TO LEARN FROM YOUR JOURNAL, READ:

Brande, Dorothea. *On Becoming a Writer* (New York: J. P. Tarcher, 1981).

Didion, Joan. "On Keeping a Notebook," in *Slouching Towards Bethlehem* (New York: Dell Publishing, 1968).

Middlebrook, Diane Wood. *Worlds into Words* (New York: W. W. Norton, 1980).

Myss, Caroline. *Anatomy of the Spirit: The Seven Stages of Power and Healing* (New York: Random House, 1996).

Myss, Caroline. *Why People Don't Heal and How They Can* (New York: Harmony Books, 1997).

Rico, Lusser Gabriele. *Writing the Natural Way* (New York: J. P. Tarcher, 1983).

Sewell, Elizabeth. *The Human Metaphor* (Notre Dame, IN: University of Notre Dame Press, 1964).

Stafford, William. "A Way of Writing," in *Writing the Australian Crawl* (Ann Arbor: University of Michigan Press, 1977).

YOU MAY ALSO CONTACT:

Shelly Carlson, Caarlsson Productions
3410-20 North Lake Shore Drive, Suite 12-I
Chicago, Illinois 60657
773-348-2421
http://www.ameritech.net/users/caarlssonproductions/
caarlssonprodcommspec.html

8.

Writing Your Authentic Self—Seven Personal Stories

Throughout this book you have learned how journal writing can guide your inner journey, promote self-discovery, and impact your life. There is no more convincing example of this than the words of those who have experienced its power. The individuals you will meet in chapter eight have been generous enough to share their true stories, their entries, and the amazing manner in which journal writing has transformed their lives. Here they are in their own words.

Shelley Grod Tatelbaum: A Healing Journal

In 1958 Shelley Grod Tatelbaum was eight years old. Her family of four included one sibling, Karen, age thirteen. Shelley and Karen were very close. They danced the jitterbug to-

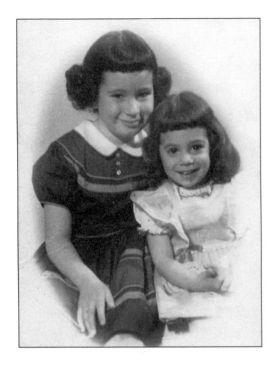

Karen and Shelley
courtesy of Shelley Tatelbaum

gether in the rec room of the family's suburban house. They pulled harmless pranks on each other and shared the joy of making music. "My favorite memory was when Karen would play the piano and I would sing. I'd pretend that I was Helen Morgan, the torch singer, and sit on the piano with a handkerchief. We would put on a concert for my parents." Karen baby-sat for her younger sister and defended her when she got into trouble with the neighborhood children. "She was my protector," says Shelley. "I was the wild kid, and she was the goody-two-shoes. There were five years between us so there wasn't much sibling rivalry. Karen was a very giving person. She was also unsure of herself. I was very sure of myself, so we balanced each other and encouraged one another."

Shelley continues, "We were a typical family which had a very untypical tragedy happen to us." Karen was diagnosed with cancer of the adrenal gland and the prognosis was grim. The doctors expected her to live only six months. Shelley says, "They told my father my sister's diagnosis on a Friday night and then on Sunday he died of a massive heart attack at the age of thirty-six. We kept my father's death from my sister until she returned from the hospital as we didn't want to add to the burden of grief in her struggle for recovery." Karen's cancer metastasized to the kidney and liver. She died seven months later.

During the period that followed these two deaths, Shelley and her mother tried to cope with the devastating losses and to find a way to live together in the new configuration of their family. For young Shelley, it was especially hard. "Remember that in those days, the 1950s, children weren't allowed to go to hospitals to visit the sick or to attend funerals. So there wasn't the kind of closure we have now in the 1990s. Also, during those years, the relationship with my mother was difficult. She was so overwhelmed with her own grief that she had little energy left for mine. Children were disenfranchised grievers back then. It was not acknowledged or sanctioned. I needed some kind of outlet so I started a journal and wrote it to my sister. I was able to connect important rituals and events of my life and share it with someone who would only listen. The power in it was that I wrote it to her. I wrote whenever I felt confused, scared, alone, or miserable. In retrospect, it was a wonderful and healthy way of healing grief—without that being my intention."

April 4, 1963

Dear Karen,

School. Frank and I broke up for good. . . . He was the only boy I ever really loved with all my heart. I have to go and do my homework. I am starting to cry again now. Help me. I do not want to talk to Mom about this. She thinks I am too young to have boyfriends anyway so she will get mad and not understand. Please come into my dreams tonight and tell me what to do. I have to go because I have so much homework. HELP!!!!!
Love, Shelley

May 20

Dear Karen,

School. Not much new there. Today makes 4 years that you died. That is really weird. I wonder what we would be doing right now if you were still alive. Mommy has not said anything about it. I did not want to tell her that I knew because I did not want to make her cry. We went to Aunt Frieda's friends for supper. I came home and did homework.
Love, Shelley

June 29

Dear Karen,

This morning we went to Grandma Mamie's unveiling. We visited Daddy Irving's grave and yours and Aunt Frieda's. It is too weird. It makes me too sad. What are you doing there anyway? I hate that you

and Daddy Irving are there and Mommy and me are left down here. I want us to be together again. I am crying now and I do not want to be soooo sad. Why did you both have to die and leave us here? . . .
Love, Shelley

September 1

Dear Karen,
. . . We went to Caldwell to see Grandma. She is going to die soon. She is pretty sick. Mommy is worried and it smells in that convalescent home. She has to sit on a tube. She is so skinny and sick looking. It makes me scared to be there and Mommy is sad. Do you think you can come to her in her dream tonight and help her? She is so sad and worried. I hate it when she gets like that. I do not want anything to happen to her. Who will take care of me if she dies? HELP.
Love, Shelley

October 18

Dear Karen,
. . . Grandma Mama died of a heart attack at about 7 P.M. Mommy's mommy. I am going to miss her but at least she is not in misery any more. Mommy is really sad. Here we go again. Everyone dies in our family. Why? Could you please tell me why. I hate this feeling in my stomach that I get whenever someone dies. What's up with that? It is a wasted day. I love you.
Love, Shelley

November 22

Dear Karen,
Guess what? President Kennedy our 35th president was assassinated today. I can't believe it. He was shot in the temple and neck in Dallas, Texas at 2 P.M. It is so sad. Everyone is shocked and crying. . . . I felt bad for his family. Everyone is shocked but me. Everyone seems to die. The father of our country and my father are together now with you. That is really weird. What do you think? Do you know who did it? I can't watch Dr. Kildare now because there is only news about the president being assassinated. Life is so stupid sometimes. They did not have it all over the news when you and Daddy died. Oh well. I love you.
Shelley

"I had two journals," says Shelley. "One was a bound book and the other was a notebook. The notebook journal was for the things I never wanted anyone to see. I used it for catharting feelings that were ugly but real. I needed to express my authentic self—get it all out—so I could process it. I used automatic writing. Then I would reread it. When I felt I had expressed all my feelings I would rip the pages out of the notebook and burn it. I would watch my pain go up in smoke."

For forty years, Shelley has been regularly writing in her journals. She writes down experiences, thoughts, and feelings, and goes back to these entries from time to time to gain a deeper understanding of what has happened in her life. Her journal is also a safe way to express a range of emotions. "It's an effective way of letting off steam," she says. "And a wonderful way of using the energy in a productive way." In raising her own two girls, Shelley encouraged her daughters to keep journals. "My daughters are diligent journal writers. I got them started by buying them diaries when they were old enough to write. Some of their journals go back to first or second grade. When they would be upset with me or life, I would say 'Go write this out in your journal!' It makes me very proud . . . for I know how valuable the experience is and how it will become even more cherished with time. It feels like we have started a family tradition. It took a tragedy for me to start to write and I am grateful that they did not need a tragedy—it is simply something they enjoy."

Shelley is now a certified grief therapist and grief educator. She holds a master's in family and pastoral therapy. She is also the founder/director of the Center for Grief, Loss and Life Transition in Poughkeepsie, New York. In her work helping clients cope with loss, Shelley has them keep journals. "When I work with my clients on issues of guilt and anger, I tell them to write it and then burn it, so the energy gets out and expressed rather than suppressed and turned inward, which leads to depression.

"Often people simply need a place to begin their healing process. Journals aid in healing grief by uncovering what is buried. They are a measurement of a journey. When we experience the pain of loss, we all want to feel better. A journal helps. It becomes a sacred text and we can measure where we've been, where we are, and where we are going as well as our dreams and fantasies."

As for Shelley, she no longer writes to her sister on a regular basis. "That stopped a long time ago. . . . I needed her when I was younger, and interestingly enough, I need her again now. I have written to her recently in journals because last year my mom was having health issues and I was feeling very alone. I wished my sister was there to help me decide things and discuss certain issues. But for the most part, now I have no need to put it in a letter format. I just write free form."

Laurine Jarvis:
A Wellness/Illness Journal

For Laurine Jarvis of Ottawa, Canada, journals provide a way to process experiences and a means to cope with chronic illness. For twenty years, she has suffered from an immune system deficiency that has led to a number of illnesses including inflammatory bowel disease, asthma, and bursitis. She writes to gain insight and to draw connections between feelings and their sources. Is she really angry in response to a relationship in her life, or are her powerful feelings actually connected to her illness? Laurine uses her journal to find out. "When you are sick, you need a lot of solitude but instead you get a lot of people around to help do things you cannot do by yourself. Then you need to manage all these people and it is a full-time job. Very tiring."

Journal writing has aided Laurine in understanding and managing her condition. "I was asked to keep symptom journals after I had been sick for a while. The first time was by a behaviorist who wanted to see if my physical symptoms were connected with my emotions. When I was first very ill I sometimes kept a symptom journal, trying to connect what foods or medications or activities might be aggravating the condition. This was actually quite helpful and even allowed me to make a chart to show my doctor, and I discovered that there were medications, activities, and foods that did, in fact, make a difference."

Regular entries give Laurine the most complete picture of her illness and access to her inner voice. "If I'm writing in a symptom journal I write throughout the day because I forget things if I don't. For other journal writing I try to write first thing in the morning before I come in contact with anyone. I find I can be in touch with my feelings easier then. I have a meditation room and I always write in my rocking chair in that room, and I have relaxing music that I play while I'm journal writing."

28 February 1999 - Sunday

new symptoms) scare me. Always have.
Not exactly sure why - maybe just
because I don't understand what's
going on. Doctor doesn't know what's
going on. Maybe I get scared because
I have to pay attention and monitor -
focus on symptoms and being sick.
Usually I stay ~~unconscious~~ until it becomes
clear what's happening or, more
often, I get used to it and don't
have to pay attention anymore. This
time I suspect my symptoms are
caused by treatment, so I'm not
just scared, I'm MAD. Somebody
should have told me the possible
side effects. How can I make choices
if I don't have all the information?
I used to be so diligent about doing
my own research that some doctors
got angry - it's MY body, MY life, MY
decision. Not a popular position I
This time I was tired and lax - trusted
too much - didn't ask enough questions.
Don't know how I'll come out of this
one but I think it could have been
prevented and that makes me SO MAD.
Who can ~~...~~ I have to be my own
doctor too? ~~...~~ are merely consultants.

Daughter and granddau~~ghter~~ come home
today - ray of sunshine. ~~...~~ is
precious and such a privileg~~e~~
around. Very crummy to feel ~~...~~

A page from Laurine Jarvis's journal
courtesy of Laurine Jarvis

Writing Your Authentic Self—Seven Personal Stories

1 March 1993—Monday

I felt centered and refreshed this morning for the first time in ages and the pain is at a minimum. What a treat! Maybe the sleeping pills help. I slept THREE HOURS straight. I can't remember the last time I slept that long at one stretch. Today I wrote letters and faxes and felt like going out. But now I'm really tired. Time to rest. The other medication I'm taking makes me hungry. I can't stop eating. I'm ready to eat dog biscuits.

With chronic illness there are ups and downs. One way Laurine copes with difficult times is by using her journal as a resource and reminder of past experiences. "I have reread entries from my symptom journals when I've become sicker and forget what to do. I see what I ate before, and what treatments I tried, what activities I engaged in, etc. It's easy to forget those things when I feel better. I seldom read other journal entries, but I have occasionally if I want to see if there's a pattern around something in particular. Usually I just keep journal writing."

Coping with a chronic illness has created conflicts for Laurine in her family life. "I started writing more about my emotions. How I felt about my illness and its impact on my life. How I felt about my kids and my inability to be with them in the ways I pictured 'normal' people being with their kids. My journals are filled with stuff about my kids. In fact, at one point I wrote "I see my journal is full of other people. Where am I?" I've been trying to focus more on me."

23 July 1998—Thursday

. . . A part of me is in denial, not believing that I'm sick at all. Part of me blames myself for being sick. If only I did this different, or that different, I wouldn't be sick. Then I think I have to act like I'm not sick because it's all my fault anyway. And part of me sees all of this, including the fact that I am sick and that the sickness isn't me. Who I am is different than what has happened to my body. . . .

Everybody's leaving me. I'd rather go with them, or at least be doing something on my own instead of staying here. The amount of help I have interferes with the solitude I yearn for and yet I don't have enough help so I'm not really taken care of, either. What I yearn for is independence. I never thought I'd be so dependent. I was always the one who helped. It's been hard adjusting to being the one who gets helped. A life lesson that's rather humbling.

25 October 1998—Sunday

A Citizen Advocacy representative was here today. Said I am a good advocate for myself, but I qualify for their programme because there is nobody in my life that isn't paid to be here. I don't have any friends. My homemaker said I could have friends if I wanted to. It's all in my attitude, she said. That really made me mad. I am basically housebound. I can't volunteer for anything, I can't attend classes, I can't get out and meet people. How would I make friends in a city I didn't live in before I became ill? It's hard to have people not understand. It's particularly hard to have people who are supposed to be caring for me be so insensitive.

"I'm not fanatic about my journal writing, but I keep fairly current," says Laurine. "Part of my illness is a kind of cognitive dysfunction. I forget things, have short-term memory loss, and although I am very articulate, I can't organize papers in chronological order and I sometimes get lost on the way home from the grocery store. I journal to clarify things in my mind. I become more centered when I journal. Sometimes I avoid journal writing because painful feelings are evoked and I don't want to feel them. Often I journal for the same reason—painful feelings come up and I want to deal with them in some way. And sometimes I journal because there are wonderful things happening that I want to remember or be reminded of."

16 February 1999—Tuesday

When good things happen I feel sad. Reminds me of all the things I can't do when I have wonderful things around me and I still feel pain and fatigue and confusion. I want to help my daughters decorate their apartments. I want to take my granddaughters out by myself. I want to have a life. I want to make a difference in the world. So many ideas, so little energy. . . .

Being sick is really the pits. I need to keep journalling so I stay centered and don't be irritable with other people just because I feel unwell. That is one of my life's challenges. Of course then I expect other people to treat me in kind and that doesn't happen too often. I'm not always as tolerant as people want me to be. It's hard to integrate all the parts of my self. I feel so enthusiastic about life. There are so many things I want to do. There are so many things I actually do. I have a very full life. . . . Mostly I'm grateful for the opportunity to learn so much. Sometimes I lose sight of

that, but in my quiet room, where I find my peace, I remember it quickly. Life is full of shattered
dreams. For all of us. I want to learn to live with it as it comes and not as I want it to be.

Laurine says, "What's powerful for me about journal writing isn't in the entries, it's the process of writing. I write until I feel free—until I'm not in reaction anymore. I then often feel prepared to cope with whatever faces me. I feel in touch with me—with the spirited self who loves life and feels joyous and creative and capable. When I've written enough that I've reached that point I stop. I've vented, I've written enough that I can put the pieces together and I don't need to write any more. I want to go do the things I've been freed up to do."

Marc Coyne: A Journal on the Inner Life of a Writer

Marc Coyne is currently a journalist in Paris. Although he intended his journals to be private, he has generously agreed to share them under this pseudonym.

Marc has been keeping journals for twelve years. He began writing at the age of sixteen in order to cope with a family crisis. He explains, "The reason I started writing is because my parents and grandparents were thinking of putting my great-grandmother in a nursing home. I couldn't understand it. I started writing about how I was feeling. It was my way of trying to control the situation. It was like giving a speech I knew I couldn't give to anyone else. This journal entry was written as a narrative because I needed to tell the story. It was cathartic and it helped me feel better." Marc ended up showing the writing to his high school teacher, who was impressed by it and encouraged Marc to continue to keep a journal.

She was old and tired and could hardly bring a glass to her lips since her wrinkled fingers trembled
so much. But she still could laugh when my brother and I wrestled. She still could say grace at hol-
idays and remember my name, at least half the time. But my parents wanted to put her away in a
nursing home, like you put an old coat you don't want any more in the attic. That coat may still be
there, but you never see it again. Never.

Ultimately, Marc's great-grandmother was moved to a nursing home. Although this was not the course of action Marc wanted, writing about his feelings was one positive thing that came out of a difficult situation. The impulse to write about his thoughts and observations continued as Marc grew. For a time, he wrote every day and documented the many details of his life. Then he found himself writing less frequently. Sometimes months would go by without a single entry, followed by a burst of expression that could go on for weeks.

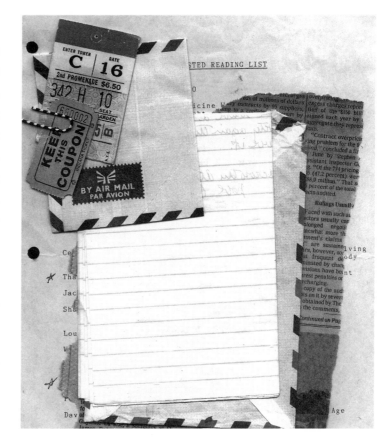

A page from Marc Coyne's journal
Courtesy of Marc Coyne

In his early journals, Marc would include keepsake objects, like articles, cards, concert tickets, and even a bracelet from a South American girl he met. For that period of time, the journals functioned much like a scrapbook of his experiences. "When I started, I was writing in a series of three-ring notebooks, mostly just stream of consciousness. Then the writing became more crafted. I switched to using a computer—my handwriting is appalling. I type 80 words per minute so my thoughts can appear on the page much more quickly and I don't have to wait for my hand to follow my thoughts. I rarely edit myself and I don't spellcheck, because it simply doesn't matter.

"I write mostly before going to bed. I write about my day. Sometimes I take themes like my love life, or a book I've read, or a movie I watched, or something I saw on the street." Once a year he prints out his entries and stores them, with his computer disks, in an old steel traveling trunk. "I'd be horrified if anything happened to them."

> *Saturday I went to Arlington Cemetery and strolled through the manicured lawns and thought*
> *of how great my country is and the sacrifices those have made for it. I also thought how pale*
> *in comparison my contributions have been so far. But mostly, I thought of the young men and*
> *women who never were given a chance, and I thought of the ridiculousness of war (and its*
> *necessity as well). I saw Kennedy's tomb and the eternal flame. The changing of the guard*
> *was magnificent, a suitable honor for those who found death while serving their country.*
> *Leaving, I was walking in front of a mom and her five-year-old daughter who asked a*
> *poignant question as a group of Korean soldiers were walking toward me; the young girl with*
> *curly black hair asked, "Mom, are there more Christians than bad people in the*
> *world?" Tough question. . . .*

Marc sees his journals as an important link to his interior life. His writings are very private. "They are not a legacy for my great-grandson, they are for me." But on occasion, he has shown his journal to others. "I wooed my first love with my journal. The second day I met her, I showed her one of the pages because I wanted to share myself. I'm not effusive with emotion, and it was my way of letting her in."

> *Entertained by young faces lighting in response to a buoyant gray-haired tour guide dancing about,*
> *"How many people do you see in this picture, What is she handing him, What are the arrows used*
> *for by Cupid? And one particularly inviting question, How do these two naked bodies look?"*
> *To the answer of a ten-year-old boy in a light blue collared shirt, "It looks like they just made*
> *love." Smiles and hidden embarrassment lingered throughout the room. I doubt the teacher expected*
> *any such answer. Throughout the gallery, stampedes of grade-school students noisily passed holding*
> *hands and peering about with abandon, minor figures but important ones gazing at the master-*
> *pieces. Funny thing was I missed Julie especially bad that afternoon.*

The journals have served Marc in his career as a professional writer. "Occasionally I've drawn from the emotions expressed in my journals to apply to the characters I'm writing about. I can almost go to the exact page and find that journal entry—whether it's about breaking up with somebody or a work issue—and apply it to my writing."

About the importance of journal writing, Marc says, "Most writers that I know have written in journals at one time or another. It helps with your writing because it loosens you up. It's practice. It's a writer's way of working out...I find it necessary. I can't see ever giving it up. I'd get lost."

Alan Leon: A Visual Journal

Alan Leon, artist and muralist living in northern California, is an avid traveler. Twenty-four years ago he made a trip to Trinidad and Tobago. "Since I was on an island I decided to study where the land and water meet because that's where things happen. I picked six places and documented these sites with writing and drawing. My goal was to open myself up to the experience of being in an unfamiliar place. I would spend the entire day sitting in one place and observing. I explored what I call 'the phenomenon of place'—all the characteristics that make a place unique. I would note schoolchildren passing, people feeding chickens, boats coming in. This got me hooked on journal writing."

Tropical smells once experienced are so vivid you easily remember when they waft across your nose again. The sweet perfume of hibiscus tinged air mixed with a breeze carrying garlic and plantain cooking together—spicy clove cigarettes saturated into brown black batik longis—fast, fetid, rankness of decaying organics becoming earth—soil—musk—savory odor of blackened bangus (fish) broiled over an open fire—passionfruit, mango, guava, pawpaw, kalamansi fruit medley.

Alan has kept journals ever since Tobago. He writes most extensively when he travels and almost daily in his journal/datebook. "The idea is to record what went on to show me where I've been in my life at a glance." He is always ready to write because his journal is with him at all times. During the day he keeps it in his shoulder bag,

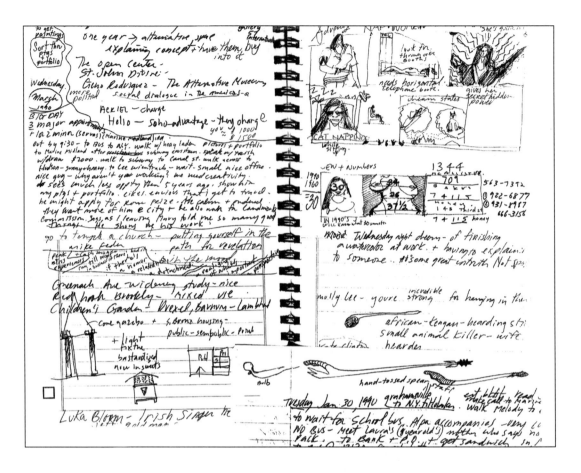

A page from Alan Leon's journal
Courtesy of Alan Leon

and at night it is by his bed. Inspiration comes at varying times. Alan says, "The muse is more likely to strike when you're ready. Sometimes I'll get up at 3:00 A.M. and I'll pour out an amazing amount of words and images."

When Alan rereads old entries, he is impressed by how the place he has visited or the experience he has had is instantly brought back by a few trigger words. "I'm often surprised in looking back at the journals at how I had that thought or did that activity. And I'm glad that there is a record of this. It's a dialogue with myself. It's a lot like meditation in that it lets me drop into my life and feel it is important. It's a way of honoring who I am."

Look at chart on wall correlating the constellations with the Nazca lines. Amazing echoes. Think about desert, colorless sandy environment as opposed to the Paracas color textiles. Love of color must be a universal. . . . Like the freedom of being my own boss—relaxing, making decisions as I care to do, not rushing, absorbing the local flavors.

It is also a way for Alan to clarify and shape his life path. "Sometimes I realize I've written about something again and again. And the more I write, the more the intention is set, the more it becomes a reality. It helps me manifest things. For example, I had written a lot about living on the West Coast years before I came here. I reread the writing now and I see the process that brought me here."

As a visual artist, the way Alan's journals look is extremely important to him. "I pick journals that are very, very beautiful and nice to hold. I've made several journals as well. Red is a color that factors in my journals a lot. Red is the color of warmth, excitement, passion, and movement. It's so beautiful to see red stitching against white pages. For the covers, I pick colors, patterns, and textures that give a feeling of a microcosm—its own little world."

The tools he uses for writing are equally important to Alan. "I have a pen collection which includes Mt. Blanc, aerodynamically shaped Italian markers, and antique fountain pens made of luminescent and pearlescent material. I use different color inks on a single page, and sometimes I use colored pencils. I love pens, though, because they are ministaffs, like a king's scepter. One of my favorite pens has a nib that one needs to dip in an inkwell. I appreciate the process and sensuality of a pen that uses ink and goes on the paper irregularly."

Alan's journals are works of art unto themselves. He describes them as "books of words liberally peppered with thumbnail sketches—literally the size of a thumbnail." The illustrations are whimsical and detailed. Often the pictures are of things he has seen, but sometimes they are diagrams or technical notes like measurements. He also includes lyrics to songs, phrases from the countries he is visiting, lists of activities, accounts of monies spent and purchases made, as well as dreams. In the borders there are titles or words highlighting sections of copy which serve as notes for future reference. In place of traditional narrative text, Alan uses short clusters of words—like poems—to capture his experiences.

Sky cloud, puff blue-gray-white hazy moire patterns, jewel dots, pink orange lining, get brighter and more intense, white silver, yellow orange, purple gold (magenta)

"I favor notebooks of odd sizes. I have a journal from Indonesia that is four inches wide and twelve inches tall. A funny shape. It's like entering an elegant tower when you open this book. I write on lined or unlined pages and the words are all over the place. Each page is a different composition—usually a mixture of text and pictures."

Alan keeps his thirty completed journals on shelves at the top of his stairs so they can be readily accessible. Every three to four weeks he revisits old writings. "I was thinking of a time when I was in Hawaii. There had just been a sudden rain. I saw a woman sitting in a particular position by a fountain and something about it reminded me of a Botticelli painting. I wrote about it. When I reread it, it makes me want to make art. It's not a concrete or sequential process really. It's a random, abstract process of inspiration. Then I take pen and paper in hand and explore the idea because of my passion for drawing."

Alex Cyril: A Young Performer's Journal

Alex Cyril is a professional performer living in Portland, Oregon. Her work has progressed from postmodern dance, to improvisation, to aerial work, specifically trapeze. Journal writing has enabled her to validate dedicating her life to being an artist and to cope with the stresses of forging a career in the performing arts.

She says, "I started writing a journal in college for an English class I was taking. I delved into the form, enjoyed it, and began using it for myself outside of class assignments. Because I was away from home, separated from my family and friends, journal writing was a way to talk to myself and figure out what I was doing. I used my writing to learn why I found myself far away from home and why I was seeking what I was seeking. I left college after a year but my journal writing continues."

The desire to focus on dance was the reason Alex left college. She embarked on a new adventure, living alone in the city for the first time and pushing against her father's vision of what her life should be. "My father had wanted me to finish school.

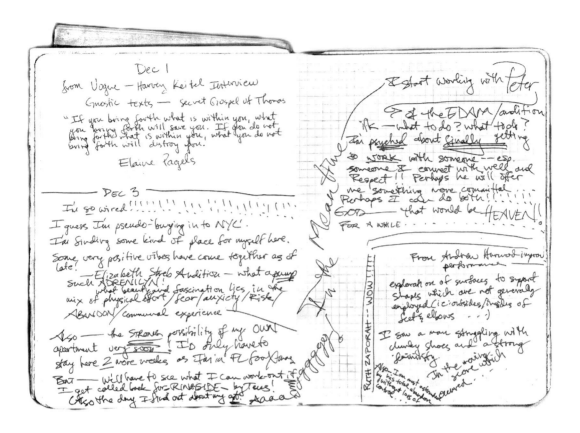

A page from Alex Cyril's journal
courtesy of Alex Cyril

When I left, we came to an understanding, but it was not his first choice for me. I was beginning to discover the hard road I'd selected in wanting to become an artist."

. . . Progress moves steadily onward and at such a rate that I begin to lose sight of how far I've come and instead look to how far I still have to go. I begin to examine this project and my abilities against other people and projects. This process I carry to extremes. I begin comparing every detail of everything unrelated and feel so overwhelmed. How could I have even thought of attempting something so monumental? I can't even see how far I've come and progress isn't progress anymore. So now I plod along on something that I don't even think I can finish and as a result the work is lacking. So I just stop working altogether and sit and watch everything I've built up to this point

fall down and crumble under the inevitable elements. I just watch knowing that I have the power to keep this from happening but unwilling to do anything about it. I'm just letting fate take its course and will let whatever happens to me happen.

"I lost my father when I was nineteen and my brother several years later," Alex continues. "I've written about pain and sorrow. I digested these feelings through my journals and put this back out through my performance. In my work, I am asked to do a lot of improvising. Sometimes a mood that I have written about in a journal will be a source. Rereading it puts me in a place to improvise from."

After the death of her father, Alex inherited insurance money. This money enabled her to continue her education in dance. The terrible irony and the price she paid for her financial independence was not lost on Alex. She wrote about it in her journal.

What worries me most is that I feel as if I cheated to become this person that I am. I feel as though it's a lie to say I've become independent and self-directed because I've been afforded this opportunity through blood money and it sickens me.

Alex has been keeping journals for thirteen years. The journals document a significant period of her life. She covers her early adult years when she entered the world and embarked on the career that her heart told her was her true path. "During the time that I decided to pursue performing I was constantly seeking venues for my dance. My journals are plagued with doubts and fears about what I was doing. Where is this going to take me now? Most of my friends or relationships were formed through pursuing my career, while others were stifled because of my constant traveling. Mixed in among the entries on dance was writing about my relationships. It was my way of coping."

I have a lot of doubts lately about the choices I've made in my life. I'm afraid of not having a purpose. I've felt that I want to dance and I love that life but maybe I love the sacrificing and outward appearance more than what I'm sacrificing for. . . . I think I'm more afraid of going home to nothing than staying here and doing something I'm not sure I want.

She has lived and danced in many cities throughout the United States, Canada, and Europe. Therefore, her journals chronicle travel experiences as well as her performances.

"I usually keep my current journal at hand as I'm working. I use it to map out choreography as well as to comment on my days," Alex says. "I used to carry my journal with me every day in my dance bag. It was a great source of information for me, a constant reference, and a way to stay connected to people I wasn't with. I would write ideas for letters to people or discussions I wanted to have when I got back from my trips. I'd also jot down ideas for stories or dance. And I referred to class dance exercises I had notated from my mentors that would facilitate my training while traveling. When I stopped doing constant traveling, I stopped carrying them with me. Getting married and buying a house gave me more permanence, and the journals are now left at home."

Dec. 1992—Germany

. . . I am still searching for my way of blending all of my experience into the productive way of life I seek. Traveling is certainly opening my mind and my soul to many new perspectives. I continue to struggle with the challenge of keeping myself motivated to dance in the solitude which traveling imposes. As soon as I begin moving, though—in class or by myself—I rediscover my passion and and am able to move forward. . . .

Dec. 1992—France

. . . The language that I most want to master, though, is movement. I understand that I will never be its master. I understand now that I've been approaching it the wrong way. I've been looking at it from the outside—on other people—and I need to find my means of communication from the inside. It is all connected to a very basic understanding. The beauty I seek, which is clarity, is revealed through simplicity. The challenge is to become complex in your statement while maintaining this clarity—perhaps by refining each expression to its simplest?

Dec. 1993—New York

. . . It's been a busy and revelatory week . . . all this activity is exactly what I've been craving and imagining for myself for many years. It's funny—I didn't see it coming, and here I am dancing in New York. I'm on the periphery of the improv community—still able to view things objectively and choose people to connect with selectively. I feel stronger than ever about maintaining my path of

integrity. Even if that means stopping dancing altogether—I can trust the discerning sense I've developed through collected experience of work from everywhere I've gone . . . .

"At first, I wrote on pages in spiral notebooks," says Alex, "then I started using more than one notebook at a time, and a freer format. Instead of grammatical sentences I'd use half sentences, poetry, and pieces of ideas."

Oct. 1994—Vancouver BC

Brisk cool air blowing into my body, through my built-up tensions—passing them off into the void behind me—I cross the bridge and the beauty of the city around me, the river under me, the air passing through me, REVIVE me—bring me back to senses I've lately strayed from. I am fulfilled here, in this power place—my Vancouver, where I keep being drawn and arriving in to positively reap bushels—Settled with myself, alive amongst women who I see eye to eye with and who help me see beyond, full in my artistry, appreciated for my skill and my dedication . . . .

"When I write, I do it from the perspective that there is an audience for my words. Who it is, I don't know. But this audience also includes myself. . . . My journal is the only place where I have brutally honest discourse. It is my psyche, my inner thoughts. I guard the giving out of this information. Once someone read a journal that was left out by accident and that was devastating. I didn't know what they had read and how that made them feel. It changed our relationship."

On the significance of journal writing in her life, Alex says, "There was a time where I needed to temporarily put my journals aside. My emotional experience was so well captured on the page, yet I wasn't experiencing it as clearly in my relationships. So I spent time rereading old entries and learned what I needed to say and how to say it directly to the people in my life. There is so much more clarity to my interpretation of old journal pages as time goes by and patterns of my actions and feelings emerge. . . . I am interested in broadening my wisdom and understanding the complexity that comes with age. This will surely be recorded on the pages of my journals. I must have made some progress on this front because the first entry upon returning to my journal was composing my marriage vows.

Perhaps the journals will be a legacy of honest self-exploration to enlighten my children some day."

William Levitt, Jr.: A Professor's Etching and Dream Journals

William Levitt, Jr., Ph.D., is an art history professor, printmaker, and antiques dealer, living in Red Hook, New York. "For me, my various professions are very related. I have always appreciated objects and feel that I learn from them. If I really love an object, it sometimes appears in my artwork. I am also interested in patterns or recurring themes. In Jungian vocabulary they would be called archetypes."

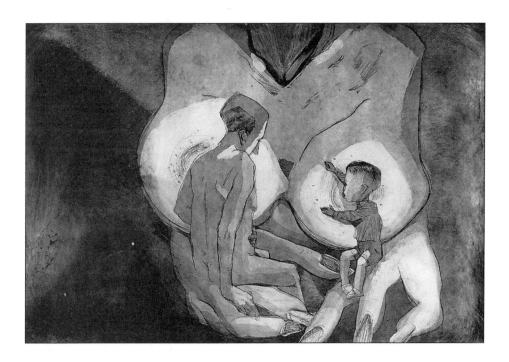

"Still Hungry," etching/aquatint by William Levitt, Jr. ©1999
courtesy of William Levitt, Jr.

The threads connecting his multifaceted career tie together in his richly layered journals. "I've kept journals most of my adult life," says William. "I was nineteen or twenty when I started and I'm now fifty-seven, so we're talking about a long period of time. I guess I began because of the need to save things. To save ideas and events. One of my teachers once told me: 'All artists are pack rats,' and I suppose this is true even with ideas and experiences. My urge to preserve may have more to do with my background as an historian."

William continues, "I don't make daily entries, it's more erratic. My journals contain a combination of dreams I've had, quotes I've read and want to save, and notes about my life. These things are important for me to include. Especially events in my life that I want to look up so I can see exactly how I felt when they occurred. It is hard to recall emotions clearly after years have passed. This way is exact."

William has discovered that it is less important for him to revisit old journal entries than to capture them on paper for preservation. "An odd thing is that I always thought I would go back and reread these journals and experience my life again, but I haven't. I go to find dreams though. Jung said that one dream in isolation has very little meaning—it is a sequence of dreams that holds the development of a theme. So I go back frequently to look up dreams for deeper understanding. My fantasy is that at some point I will reread the entire series of journals, but that hasn't happened yet.

"I keep two journals. One is for dreams, the other is for the series of etchings I'm working on. The etching journals track the genesis of each image and the metamorphosis of them as well. I write about the meaning of each image I create. Each image has a visible subject, but for me there is a subtext and an emotional or implied subject. This may differ very much from what you see on the surface in the same way that a Renaissance painting of the holy family may have as its actual subject the new science of perspective or anatomy. The surface subject and the actual subject differ. I discover, in the process of working, the implied content of the image and record that in the journal."

The series of etchings that William is creating began in 1990. The subject of this work is his complicated and symbiotic relationship with his mother, Jane. "It traces my mother's life, as a young girl, a woman, and an old woman, and my own life at various stages. The work and the writings are, for me, a form of advanced therapy. When I set out I wanted to understand. Empathy and forgiveness is more the target now."

AN ENTRY IN THE ETCHING JOURNAL

October 26, 1990

Last night's dream:
In a basement or cave I was trying to pry off the lid of Jane's coffin with hammer and crow bar. The coffin was lying on the ground. Suddenly the end to my left—the foot end—popped or slid up, a surprise as I was working on the top. Inside I saw black (as though burned) stacks of papers or books.

A woman stuck her head through the doorway from the next room and I said to her, "Tell Jane I've got it open."

Interpretation of the Dream:
And what is her actual body: blackened, scorched papers and books: ideas, not blood or heart or flesh? Her highest value I finally realized (am I being fair?) was how things looked to others. In her actual life her ideas/ideals hadn't worked for her (they blackened) and she was miserable . . . certainly this has a different feel from all those years of "talk" therapy, which left her image ambiguous for me. The therapist's idea of her sounded logical, but I couldn't feel it. These images are more equivocable than his: some positive, some negative, admiring, condemning, loving, hating— more like reality. And the principle of enantiadromia constantly works at balance: this is what produces these shifts of view as well as style, moving from tragic to comic, classic to expressive, linear to painterly. How could I reduce a living human being to a line or two? And can anyone get far enough away from his own mother to find a clear view?

William has found that participating in a dream group is extremely helpful in figuring out the meaning of a dream. Members of the group, even someone untrained, may say something useful or reveal an insight that he wouldn't have come to on his own. "A journal is indispensable for dream work. Dreams are like sea foam, they easily dissolve. I have found that it is very important to write down a dream, especially when it is fresh. When I share a dream, I read from my journal. I've found that as time passes, I may forget details if they aren't preserved in writing. Also when I work alone in trying to figure out the symbols or meaning of a dream, I work from the written records of my dreams. The act of writing it down aids me in recovering more of the dream itself."

AN ENTRY FROM THE DREAM JOURNAL

March 4, 1998, 7:55 A.M.

Last night's dream:
A number of identical young men were working for a doctor. The problem was that they all had an extremely limited range of motion. Each young man had his own compartment in a matrix of chrome-covered metal piping that fanned out like a root system and resembled auto exhaust pipes. Each was attached at his base—that is, at his feet, by a hinge, so that all he could do was rock back and forth. And for even this motion to be possible it was first necessary for an old, familiar song to be played (a recording), and for it to continue playing while they moved.

5:00 P.M.

Interpretations of the dream:
It seems clear to me—perhaps even during the dream—that the "doctor" and the "number of identical young men" are me. They are attached by their "bases, that is feet," so they cannot walk or move about; they can only "rock back and forth," stuck to home plate, as it were, incapable of independent movement. In fact each one is a kind of cell, or compartment of the pipe system, much like a single space in a spider's web.

And since the pipe system reminds me of the exhaust system of a car, it may well be a pun: the "exhausted," the system (mine) which doesn't work anymore, that is stuck, swinging in place to an "old song," the only thing which keeps it going. The "young men" are also like flies or insects caught in a spider's web, swinging to try to escape.

Aside from sharing his dream writings with others, what does he envision might happen with his years of journals well into the future? William says, "There seems to be an interest in artists' journals. I know I always find other artists' journals to be fascinating. Delacroix and Max Beckman kept journals. There were also Van Gogh's journals and letters, and Henry Moore was an amazing writer about his work. It has occurred to me that if I was successful in worldly terms, I, or someone else, would someday publish my journals."

Maria Marewski:
A Journal of Personal History

Maria Marewski, a filmmaker and the director of the Children's Media Project in Poughkeepsie, New York, received her mother's private journals after her death as well as a birthday journal written for her by her mother.

"My mother, Irmgard Just Marewski, kept diaries and journals her whole life. When she came from Germany to America at the age of thirty-six, she felt like an outsider in her new country. There was no one she could really connect with; therefore, her journal was her lifeline. I remember always seeing her writing in a black-and-white school composition book. Her private journal was a retrospective account of the time she had spent in a concentration camp as a German Catholic during World War II. In those days people didn't go to therapy, so she wrote her account as a way of processing her experience."

ENTRIES FROM IRMGARD JUST MAREWSKI'S
CONCENTRATION CAMP JOURNAL

All this suffering—our only hope was that we could endure. Every day there were new prisoners arriving. It was always a shock for us to see the faces of the new victims as they were brought into the camp. Sometimes we held our heads in disbelief. How was something like this possible? And there was no one to help. The entire country seemed to be in a trance. The only thing left for us to do was wait for the help of outsiders. . . .

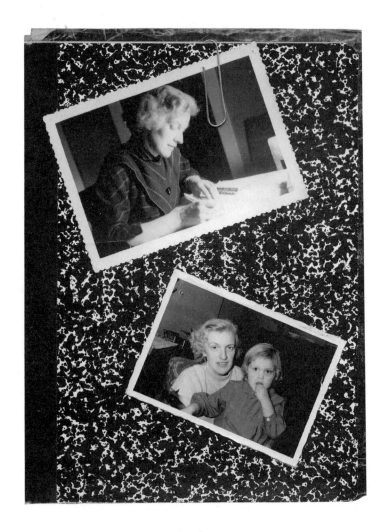

Irmgard and Maria
courtesy of Maria Marewski

It was the not knowing, the endless days of waiting and not knowing that was the most difficult. We were stuck. All we could do was wait. One of us has been here a year already without knowing why she is here. She is supposed to have expressed something punishable, but she is not aware of what her crime is. . . .

It was the same for all of us. We all suffered the same, but no one wanted to express it. We knew we would become closer if we talked about our sufferings and shared our problems. But no one wanted to get that close. Maybe it would have made our suffering worse. And so we pushed

our sorrows into a small corner of our heart and listened instead to all the stories of a better time.
In this way, all of us played a little theatre for ourselves. . . .

I marked each day on the wall of the cell. Six vertical lines and one diagonal. How many
would it be for me, and how many others had already suffered here? The scribbled prison walls
spoke volumes. I remember one such scribbling in particular. It said, "the real heroes are those who
can smile under their tears and forget their own sufferings to help others." There was also a mes-
sage on the walls from my own imprisonment. "Learn to suffer without complaining."
I scratched it on the wall with my hairpin. . . .

"The psychological trauma induced by war can have long-range effects on a family," explains Maria. "Even if the second generation has not directly experienced the
war, children inevitably absorb the emotions of their parents. . . . This unprocessed,
unhealed trauma is like the phantom pain of an amputated limb. In a way, my
mother's journal entries served to describe to me what kind of limb it was so that I
can understand how to process it."

Irmgard also wrote journals for each of her three daughters simultaneously.
The writings were an account of the girls' lives from birth to age sixteen. She
wrote frequently when they were small, less often as they grew older. She divided the
books into three areas: early childhood, childhood after emigrating to America, and
the teenage years. When they reached the age of sixteen, she stopped writing to them
because she had less access to their private lives. She presented the books to each
daughter when they turned twenty-one.

Maria believes that her mother wrote with dual motivations: for her own emotional survival and to provide a gift for her children. "My mother felt childhood was
a magical time and it was her job to witness it for us. Later, as I approached adulthood, the fact that she knew she was dying of cancer gave it more urgency. She knew
that she wouldn't be around to tell us the stories."

A BIRTHDAY JOURNAL ENTRY FROM IRMGARD TO MARIA, 1957

As Papa wanted to go away yesterday you looked at him, asking: please don't lock the door. And
Papa did not lock the door. But when he came back, what a surprise! You had been in the closet for

shoes. And you had taken all the shoes out and were working on them with shoe cream. The left-over shoe cream you put on the walls. When Papa came home, you were smiling over your whole face and showing with pride what you did.

Irmgard died the same year Maria received her birthday journal. The book was mailed because she was too weak to travel and could not deliver it in person. The journal pages were bound and had an opening page with a quotation. The quote was an important life message from Irmgard, a form of religious affirmation. Maria's quote read: "Seek ye first the kingdom of heaven and all things will be yours." Maria also received a banner of the quotation as part of her twenty-first birthday present.

Maria has been inspired by her mother's writing and used the journals as a major element in her film *In the Name of the Father*. The film's narrative voice speaks words from her mother's writing. Maria explains, "I have used my mother's journals to make sense of my own life and to process my childhood. I used them as a reality check. My mother believed, and this was clear from her concentration camp diaries, that it was important to be hopeful and optimistic," as in this entry:

ENTRY FROM IRMGARD'S
CONCENTRATION CAMP JOURNALS

I remember my 25th birthday in the camp. Everything seemed so dim and so desperate. We didn't know it then, but this was just before we were liberated. We believed then that once we were freed this nightmare would be over and we would witness a new time. A time of peace, freedom, and love. There would be no more mutilation. What we sought was a new aware-ness. What we wanted was to open the eyes of others. For all that we had been through, we came to realize that it is not dying that is tragic—but to live, without seeing what can be—this is a tragedy.

Maria continues, "As for the journals she wrote for us, at the stage of life when you are becoming an adult it is important to believe that everything is possible. Her writing was especially significant for me because from age twenty-one on she was not physically there for me, but the journal was. She couldn't give her children a sheltered childhood, but she formed me and my sisters into self-reflective people."

A BIRTHDAY JOURNAL ENTRY
FROM IRMGARD TO MARIA, 1957

I am catching myself thinking how you will develop and how your life will be. It is not easy for a mother to know that her child will also have to suffer and we cannot help you. We can only do one thing. We can educate you so you are able to stand pain and suffering.

Maria continues to record her family history by creating records for her own two children. She is using video to document their lives and plans to assemble the footage as her gift to them.

Conclusion

Remember that your journal is a journey, a path to finding your authentic self. For Maria and Irmgard, Shelley, Laurine, Marc, Alan, Alex, and William, journal writing has enhanced their capacity to cope with daily challenges, to celebrate life's joys, and to powerfully express their own voices. It can do the same for you.

Like others before you, you will discover that this is one of life's most exciting voyages, and you will be guided by your own unique perspective, style, and goals. Let the wisdom of your inner voice lead you as you record and explore your life through writing. As a result, you may access your potential, actualize your talents, and activate your authentic self as never before.

So now embark. Embark on a journey of revelation and growth as you close this book, open your own, and launch what is literally a new chapter in your life recorded on the first page of your journal.

RESOURCES

For additional examples and information on journals and how journal writing has helped people achieve transformation, check the following Web sites:

www.writerswrite.com/journal

www.dir.yahoo.com/social-science/Communications/Writing/ Journals-and-Diaries

Also note that journal sites are added to the Internet regularly. To access the latest information, type in "journal writing" or "diaries."

For information on tapes of journals read aloud, including those of some well-known historical figures, contact the Spoken Word at www.spoken-word.com

You may also check your local newspaper, library, adult education, community service, and other organizations to see if they have journal-writing classes or groups. You could even start one yourself!

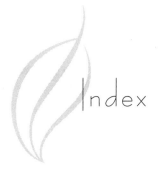

Index

A

Acorn theory, 100

Adams, Abigail, 3

Adams, Kathleen, 73, 76

Affirmations, 21, 57, 62

Aging process, 91

Alcott, Louisa May, 28, 30

All God's Children Need Traveling Shoes (Angelou), 103

Alliteration, 121

Alls' Well That Ends Well (Shakespeare), 8

Alphapoems, 73

Analyzing journal writing, 115–132

    connection between emotional and physical health, 129–131

    by dreams, 123–128

    by imagery, 118–121

    by lists, 122

    resources on, 131–132

    setbacks and reaction to change, 117–118

    by word clusters, 122–123

Anatomical photo-collage, 92

Angelou, Maya, 103

Anger, 4, 53–54

Anthony and Cleopatra (Shakespeare), 4

Aquarian Conspiracy, The (Ferguson), 118

Aquinas, Thomas, 108

Archetypal approach to journal writing, 83–84

Artist's Date, 81

Artist's Way, The, A Spiritual Path to Higher Creativity (Cameron), 79

Assonance, 121

At a Journal Workshop: Writing to Access the Power of the Unconscious and Evoke Creative Ability (Progoff), 90, 107–108

Atwood, Margaret, 53

Augustine, St., 101

Authentic self, concept of, 1

Autobiographic voice, 98–101, 105–107

Automatic writing, 55

B

Balanced information, 27, 28

Baldwin, Christina, 3, 6, 34, 78, 89

Bashkirtseff, Maria, 14

Beckman, Max, 157

Beecher, Henry Ward, 37

Benefits of journal writing, 18–35

    clarity, 19–22

    personal growth, wisdom, and maturity, 34–35

    perspective, 29–32

    problem-solving abilities, 32–33

    self-knowledge, 28–29

    trust, 24–27

    truth, 22–24

Birthday journal, 50–51

Bond Between Women, The, A Journey to Fierce Compassion (Galland), 9, 95

Branthoover, Jennifer, 32

Breathing exercise, 10

Bredenberg, Ingrid, 57

Broffman, Kary, 129, 130

Browning, Elizabeth Barrett, 40, 48

Browning, Robert, 48

Burns, Ken, 7, 109

C

Cameron, Julia, 21, 26, 27, 79–81, 98

Campbell, Don, 72

Cancer patients, 41

Career journal, 61–63

Carlson, Ruth Larson, 37–38

Carlson, Shelley, 70, 106, 118, 132

Chapman, Joyce, 86, 122

Chestnut, Mary, 7

Childhood messages, identifying, 44

Civil War, The (documentary), 7

Clarity, as benefit of journal writing, 19–22

Cleopatra, 3, 4

Clewer, Lisa Ray, 46

sample entries, 11–16
spiritual autobiography, 93–95
story/character approach to, 81–82
topics for (*see* Topics for journal writing)
writing environment, 68–69
writing instruments, 66–68
Jungian therapists, 77–78

K

Kahn, Hazrat Inayat, 15, 21
Kant, Immanuel, 108
Keller, Helen, 102
Kelsey, Morton, 78
Kitzis, Eileen, 55
Klein, Janice, 67
Kollwïtz, Kathe, 11, 14
Kravetz, Carol, 79
Krishnamurti, J., 1
Kübler-Ross, Elisabeth, 41

L

Leon, Alan, 145–148
Leonard, Linda Schierse, 62, 85
Letter-writing approach, 86–88
Levitt, William, Jr., 153–157
Lewis, C. Day, 115
Lewis, Mary, 71, 75
Life dreams, 19–22
Life of One's Own, A (Field), 14
Lists, 122
Lives of the Saints, The, 101
Location memoir, 103
Longing for Darkness: Tara and the Black Madonna (Galland), 38
Love, as topic for journal, 48–50

M

Maisel, Eric, 109
Marewski, Irmgard Just, 157–161
Marewski, Maria, 157–161
Maturity, as benefit of journal writing, 34–35
Memoirs, 102–104

Memory fragment worksheets, 124
Mental distractions, eliminating, 69
Merton, Thomas, 112
Metaphor, 121
Metcalf, Linda Trichter, 72
Metzger, Deena, 81–82, 119
Milestone letters, 86
Milestones, 85–86
Mindfulness, 75
Montaigne, Michel de, 108
Moore, Henry, 157
Moore, Thomas, 52
Morning Pages, 80
Mozart Effect, The (Campbell), 72
Music, 72
Myers, Susan Spritz, 5, 8, 17
Myss, Caroline, 117, 118, 131

N

Native American tradition, 111
Nature, as topic of journal, 38–40
Nin, Anaïs, 3, 7, 22, 102

O

Occupational memoir, 103–104
"Oh wow!" collection, 55, 56
O'Kane, Atum, 27, 30, 59
One to One: Self-Understanding Through Journal Writing (Baldwin), 34
Onomatopoeia, 121
Orman, Suze, 60
Orthodox churches, 23

P

Paine, Thomas, 108
Painter, Charlotte, 12
Pardo, Ann, 20
Parenthood, journal writing and, 49–50
Pascal, Blaise, 108
Pearson, Carol S., 25, 28, 31, 80, 83

Pennebaker, James, 42
Pepys, Samuel, 3, 108
Personal growth, journal writing and, 34–35
Personal history journal, 157–161
Personal stories, 133–161
  healing journal, 133–138
  inner life of writer, 142–145
  personal history journal, 157–161
  professor's etching and dream journals, 153–157
  visual journal, 145–148
  wellness/illness journal, 138–142
  young performer's journal, 148–153
Perspective, as benefit of journal writing, 29–32
Physical approach, 91–93
Picasso, Pablo, 102
Plummer, George Winslow, 4
Poetic Image, The (Lewis), 115
Polo, Marco, 3, 4
Prewriting, 101
Privacy, 2, 6–7, 68, 89
Problem-solving abilities, journal writing and, 32–33
Progoff, Ira, 78, 90, 107–108
Proprioceptive Writing, 72, 74
Ptolemy, 3
Pyrdek, Loretta, 71–72

R

Ranier, Tristine, 98, 100, 105
Reframing, 93
Relationship memoir, 103
Relatives, interviewing, 46–47
Release letters, 86–87
Religions, 23
Resources, 16–17, 35, 76, 96–97, 162
  on journal topics, 64–65
  on voice, 113–114

Responsibility, 11
Returning (Wakefield), 93, 94
Revelation of St. John the Divine, The, 101
Rico, Lusser Gabriele, 122, 123
Rollins, Betty, 3
Roots (Haley), 45
Rousseau, Jean-Jacques, 101–102, 108

S

Sacred pampering, 92, 130
Sand, George, 13
Santamaria, Frances Karlen, 12
Sarton, May, 23, 33
Scarf, Maggie, 24, 44, 102
Schiller, Friedrich von, 108
Schoeneck, Theresa S., 88
Scott-Maxwell, Florida, 11, 29
Scovel, Carl, 94
Secular Journal (Merton), 112
Self-censorship, 116
Self-confidence, 26
Self-criticism, 26–28
Self-judgments, 23, 26
Self-knowledge, as benefit of journal writing, 28–29
Self-portrait, 71–72
Senesh, Hannah, 13
Setbacks, analyzing, 117–118
Shah, Idries, 22, 26
Shakespeare, William, 4, 8
Sher, Barbara, 19, 21, 22, 33, 62, 78
Silence, stages of, 34
Simile, 121
Simon, Tobin, 72, 74
Simonton family, 41–42
Sketch of the Past, A (Woolf), 107
Spiritual autobiography, 93–95
Spiritual Dimensions of Psychology (Khan), 15
Spirituality, 14, 41, 58–60
Stafford, William, 15
Story/character approach to journal writing, 81–82

Story Circle Journal, 85
Story of My Life, The (Keller), 102
Story of Your Life, The: Writing a Spiritual Autobiography (Wakefield), 93
"Support Your Local Genius Night," 19
Swift, Jonathan, 108

T

Tagore, Rabindranath, 25
Tatelbaum, Shelley Grod, 89, 133–138
Taylor, Judith, 70, 75
Thank-you letters, 87–88
Thomas, Caroline, 25, 35
Thomas, Sandra, 4, 54
Thoreau, Henry David, 108
Tibetan Buddhism, 23
Tolstoy, Sophie, 12
Topics for journal, 11–14, 36–65
   birthdays, 50–51
   career, 61–63
   daily log, 37–38
   family history, 3, 43–47
   friendships, 552
   love, 48–50
   milestones, 85–86
   nature, 38–40
   resources on, 64–65
   specific emotions, 52–54
   spiritual journey, 58–60
   visual journal, 55–58
   wellness/illness, 40–43
Treasure Map, 57, 58
Trust, as benefit of journal writing, 24–27
Truth, as benefit of journal writing, 22–24

U

Understanding, Coping, and Growing Through Grief (Schoeneck), 88
United States: Essays 1952-1992 (Vidal), 108–109

V

Validation, 20
Van Gogh, Vincent, 157
Vidal, Gore, 108–109
Visual Guide, 108
Visual journal, 55–58, 145–148
Vocational memoir, 103
Vogler, Christopher, 82
Voice, 98–114
   acting exercise to find, 106
   autobiographic, 98–101 105–107
   confessional, 101–102
   fairy tales, 104–105
   of historical perspective, 109
   of humankind, 107–110
   memoirs, 102–104
   resources on, 113–114
   spiritual, 110–113

W

Wakefield, Dan, 80, 93–94
Warhol, Andy, 3
Wellness/illness journal, 40–43, 138–142
Wild Mind, Living the Writer's Life (Goldberg), 78–79
Wild Woman archetype, 84
Wimala, Bhante Y., 112
Wisdom, as benefit of journal writing, 34–35
Wisdom letters, 87
Wittig Albert, Susan, 85, 86, 99
Woolf, Virginia, 7, 9, 107
Word clusters, analyzing journal by, 122–123
Wordsworth, William, 13
World Wide Web, 35
Writing environment, 68–69
Writing instruments, 66–68
Writing the Australian Crawl (Stafford), 15